Neuromuscular Diseases during Development

Fondazione Pierfranco e Luisa Mariani
viale Bianca Maria, 28
20129 Milan, Italy

Telephone: +39 (2) 795458 & 796356
Fax: +39 (2) 76009582

NEUROMUSCULAR DISEASES DURING DEVELOPMENT

Postgraduate Course of the Pierfranco and Luisa Mariani Foundation, Milan
Collegio Borromeo, Pavia, 8–10 March 1995

Edited by
Fernando Cornelio
Giovanni Lanzi
Ermellina Fedrizzi

Mariani Foundation Paediatric Neurology Series: 5
Series editor: Maria Majno

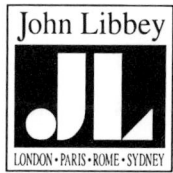

British Library Cataloguing in Publication Data

Neuromuscular diseases during development
1. Diseases
   Mariani Foundation Paediatric Neurology Series: Vol. 5
   I. Cornelio, F., Lanzi, G. and Fedrizzi, E. II. Series

ISSN: 0969–0301
ISBN: 0 86196 541 8

Published by

John Libbey & Company Ltd, 13 Smiths Yard, Summerley Street, London SW18 4HR, England
Telephone: +181–947 2777 Fax: +181–947 2664
John Libbey Eurotext Ltd, 127 Avenue de la République, 92120 Montrouge, France
John Libbey – C.I.C. s.r.l., via Lazzaro Spallanzani 11, 00161 Rome, Italy
John Libbey & Company Pty Ltd, Level 10, 15/17 Young Street, Sydney, NSW, 2000, Australia
© 1997 John Libbey & Company Ltd. All rights reserved.
Unauthorised duplication contravenes applicable laws.

Printed in Great Britain by WBC Bookbinders Ltd, Unit 5, Waterton Industrial Estate, Bridgend, Mid Glamorgan, CF13 3YN

Contents

	Preface *Ferdinando Cornelio*	vii
Chapter 1	Metabolic myopathies: general aspects and clinical approach *Edvige Veneselli*	1
Chapter 2	Clinical heterogeneity of the respiratory chain defects *Enrico Bertini, Serenella Servidei, Enzo Ricci, Gabriella Silvestri,* *Carlo Dionisi Vici, Carlo Piantadosi and Pietro Tonali*	9
Chapter 3	Congenital muscular dystrophies *Michel Fardeau, Fernando M.S. Tomé, Anne Helbling-Leclerc,* *Teresinha Evangelista, Emilia Manole, Alberto Ottolini,* *Martine Chevallay, Sabine Fauré and Dominique Hillaire*	23
Chapter 4	Dystrophinopathies *Lucia Morandi, Marina Mora, Claudia Di Blasi, Rita Barresi* *and Valeria Confalonieri*	31
Chapter 5	The congenital myopathies *Carlo P. Trevisan*	37
Chapter 6	The hereditary myotonic syndromes *Antonio Pizzuti, Giuseppe Novelli and Bruno Dallapiccola*	47
Chapter 7	Hereditary motor and sensory neuropathy (HMSN) and tomaculous neuropathy (HNPP) *Angelo Sghirlanzoni and Davide Pareyson*	57
Chapter 8	Spinal muscular atrophy: history and personal observations *Giovanni Lanzi, Angela Berardinelli and Andrea Gemma*	67
Chapter 9	Disorders of neuromuscular transmission in childhood *Paolo Confalonieri, Carlo Antozzi, Marina Mora and Renato Mantegazza*	77

Chapter 10	Current concepts review on the orthopaedic treatment of muscular diseases in childhood *Francesco Motta and Sergio Monforte*	89
Chapter 11	Therapy of scoliosis in neuromuscular pathology *André J. Kaelin*	95
Chapter 12	Respiratory pathophysiological bases for mechanical ventilation in neuromuscular diseases *Isa Cerveri, Francesco Fanfulla and Maria Cristina Zoia*	103
Chapter 13	Home mechanical ventilation and Duchenne's muscular dystrophy *Jean-Claude Raphael*	113
Chapter 14	Genetic counselling in neuromuscular disorders *Gian Antonio Danieli and Maria Luisa Mostacciuolo*	123
Chapter 15	Molecular prenatal diagnosis of neuromuscular disorders *Bruno Dallapiccola, Francesca Capon, Massimo Gennarelli, Isabella Torrente, Rita Mingarelli and Giuseppe Novelli*	131
Conclusions	The provision of global care for the patient with neuromuscular disease and his family *Giovanni Lanzi*	145
	Subject Index	151

Preface

Ferdinando Cornelio

Department of Neuromuscular Diseases, National Neurological Institute 'Carlo Besta', Via Celoria 11, 20133 Milan, Italy

This updating course on neuromuscular diseases during development took place at an opportune and auspicious time, given the spectacular growth of our understanding in this important disease area, and the consequent promise of new ways of preventing and treating neuromuscular illnesses.

The course concentrated on three main areas: the impact of molecular biology and molecular genetics on ætiology, advances in our understanding of the pathogenesis of neuromuscular diseases, and finally therapy.

Aetiological aspects were fully covered in a series of contributions in which the remarkable impact of the new molecular methodologies became fully apparent. Diagnosis and, as a consequence, clinical practice, are undergoing profound change following the growth of our understanding in this area. For example, it has now become clear that the muscular dystrophies arise from well-defined genetic defects. The defective genes in question result in altered expression or lack of expression of proteins in the plasma membrane of myofibres. Such proteins include dystrophin, whose alteration or absence give rise to the dystrophinopathies: Becker's and Duchenne's muscular dystrophy, and other conditions with milder phenotypes. Various other glycoproteins associated with dystrophin, which anchor the myofibres to the connective tissue support, may be genetically missing or altered, and these defects give rise to conditions known as limb girdle dystrophy and congenital dystrophies. The common denominator of the dystrophies is degeneration of muscle fibres and consequent fibrosis – a relationship between genotype and phenotype that remains intriguing.

A entirely new chapter on the myopathies was added with the discovery of defects in ion-channel proteins. These defects lead to a spectrum of clinical syndromes ranging from the myotonias to the so-called periodic paralyses. Molecular characterization of the defective proteins has enlightened not only the pathophysiology of these rare and interesting afflictions, but again may be expected to lead to new therapies.

The congenital structural myopathies are of special concern to the neuropaediatrician, and here too there have been some interesting developments: for example, the discovery that a defect in the ryanodine receptor is responsible for central core myopathy – a congenital form that is not altogether rare. Malignant hyperthermia, a life-threatening condition that only manifests itself during general anaesthesia, can also be associated with central core disease.

The metabolic myopathies are another important group of neuromuscular illnesses affecting children of developmental age. The various forms, whose pathological and clinical manifestations overlap, have now been well defined from the genetic and pathophysiological points of view; and in some cases adequate therapies are now available. The speakers who dealt with the metabolic myopathies provided an illuminating outline of the clinical, pathological, biochemical and genetic characteristics of these diseases. The presentation on diagnosis was especially useful, since it provided indications to alert both clinician and ultraspecialist to the possible presence of a metabolic condition in a given patient. The information given on the treatment and prevention of these important and unfortunately frequent diseases of infancy was equally helpful.

A series of generally autosomal-dominant inherited conditions, including myotonic dystrophy and Huntington's disease, have been shown by recent genetic research to be associated with so-called DNA instability. Defective DNA replication results in the elongation of certain repeat sequences of trinucleotides. The prototype neuromuscular disease of this group is myotonic dystrophy, sometimes known as Steinert's disease. Genetic analysis is able to identify the presence of the unstable repeat sequence at the locus of the gene responsible for the disease, and hence diagnose the disease. More important, however, is the fact that the length of the repeat sequence correlates with the severity of the phenotype, and this has major implications for prognosis and prevention. Several other hereditary neuropathies have been associated with the presence of unstable trinucleotide repeats.

The course provided a comprehensive update of clinical aspects of spinal muscular atrophy; here again a primary genetic defect has been discovered, at least in the majority of cases, and is it thought that two genes are involved: one responsible for the full development of motor neurons and the other for their apoptosis.

Several neuromuscular diseases in developing children are not congenital but acquired, and among the most important of these are autoimmune conditions affecting peripheral nerve or neuromuscular junction. For these conditions, new knowledge has permitted more refined diagnoses; while better understanding of the pathogenetic mechanisms has resulted in important advances in therapy: we now have available a series of treatment protocols which offer improved quality of life for sufferers of these diseases.

The final part of the course was concentrated mainly on therapy. As Professor Michael Brooke, who introduced this section, took pains to emphasize, apart from some of the metabolic and autoimmune conditions, the drugs currently available to combat neuromuscular illnesses are of little concrete value. Attention therefore mainly focused on rehabilitation, orthopaedic devices and surgery. The utility of an interdisciplinary approach to the young invalid with progressive neuromuscular disease was highlighted: specialists from several disciplines should be involved, under the overall direction of the neuropaediatrician.

Orthopaedic devices and rehabilitation techniques often allow patients to maintain their personal autonomy. But these means should always be used in such a way as to enable the patient to integrate as normally as possible with others. When autonomy is severely compromised, it is important that the patient's existence should be made as comfortable as possible, particularly when, as in the majority of cases, respiratory function is compromised. In fact, the utility of assisted ventilation was vigorously debated during the course, and the question of whether such interventions have a positive influence on autonomy or survival remains unresolved.

The tremendous impact of genetics on neuromuscular diseases became evident once more when the subject of prevention was discussed. The reliability and precision of genetic tests, and the fact that they are relatively simple to perform in a hospital laboratory, has rendered medical genetics one of the most potent diagnostic instruments available to modern medicine; this is particularly true for neuromuscular diseases of developmental age. It is imperative therefore that the neuropaediatrician is fully conversant with these techniques: a fundamental point that was the *leitmotif* of the course.

Although the identification of genetic defects is crucial for any disease prevention programme, the increasing power of genetic diagnosis may in fact render patient management more difficult, since it engenders hope of an early cure or more effective treatment; when those hopes are not realized, the repercussions on the patient can be severe. Equally, family members should not be fed false hopes, but instead should be kept judiciously informed: most young patients with neuromuscular diseases become severely disabled and will require continuing dedication and help from their family.

Another aspect of the problem is the impact of medical genetics on society as a whole. The availability of new and sophisticated genetic tests can lead to increased expectations with regard to therapy and, on the other hand, a mistaken allocation of resources. Here the clinician has a fundamental role: to establish a relationship with the patient, to weigh up what technology can offer the patient and his family, and to counsel the family about prevention, treatment and everything else concerning the future of the young patient. All these points were eloquently emphasized by Professor Lanzi in his concluding remarks.

In conclusion, the course could not cover all new developments in neuromuscular diseases, but it had the merit of presenting objective and comprehensive contributions from major figures in the field. The clinicians and health professionals who attended had the benefit of a wide-ranging and competent update that will undoubtedly help them in their day-to-day contact with young neuromuscular patients.

Chapter 1

Metabolic myopathies: general aspects and clinical approach

Edvige Veneselli

Department of Child Neuropsychiatry, G. Gaslini Institute, University of Genoa, 16147 Genoa, Italy

Summary

Metabolic myopathies are a group of clinically heterogeneous myopathies, defined by the detection of a specific biochemical anomaly.

They can be subdivided into glycogenolytic and glycolytic disorders, myopathies due to transport and fatty acid oxidation defects, mitochondrial myopathies and myopathies due to altered purine metabolism.

The clinical approach includes a preliminary investigation entailing family history, age at onset, muscular involvement, and muscular appearance either isolated or in association with involvement of the heart, liver, CNS and other organs.

The main clinical pictures suggesting a metabolic ætiology are examined. Laboratory investigations are differentiated in relation to the characteristics observed: the diagnostic procedures are quite limited in some forms of glycogenosis, but are complex in others, e.g. multisystemic mitochondrial diseases.

A therapeutic approach is possible in several diseases, and is sometimes successful, as in carnitine deficiency.

Prenatal diagnosis is possible in forms with known enzyme deficiency or with identified genetic markers.

Metabolic myopathies are a group of clinically heterogeneous disorders, characterized by a specific biochemical anomaly. They can be subdivided into the following sub-groups: disorders of glycogenolysis and glycolysis (glycogenoses), myopathies due to lipid transport and oxidation defects, mitochondrial myopathies and myopathies due to altered purine metabolism. They are a group of inborn errors of intermediary metabolism with symptoms often due to a deficiency in energy production or utilization, occurring in the muscle but also in other energy-consuming organs such as the heart, the liver and the brain.

Metabolic myopathies have been widely examined in the literature (De Vivo, 1993; Di Donato, 1994; Di Mauro & Tsujino, 1994; Saudubray & Charpentier, 1995). After some brief introductory remarks, this Chapter will focus attention on the clinical approach as the most appropriate procedure to identify adequate and effective diagnostic methods.

Muscular glycogenoses (GSD) (Engel & Hirschhorn, 1994; Di Mauro & Tsujino, 1994; Dubowitz, 1995; Brumback *et al.*, 1992) present two principal clinical pictures. In infancy and childhood, progressive myopathy appears above all as GSD type II or Pompe's disease due to acid maltase deficiency, GSD type III or Cori's disease due to debrancher enzyme deficit (amylo-1,6-glucosidase), and GSD type IV or Andersen's disease due to branching enzyme deficit (amylo-1,4–1,6-transglucosidase).

In childhood and adolescence, exercise intolerance and painful contractures, sometimes with myoglobinuria, occur in GSD type V or McArdle's disease, due to muscular phosphorylase deficiency, GSD type VII or Tarui's disease due to deficiency of fructokinase, and also phosphorylase b kinase, phosphoglycerate kinase, phosphoglycerate mutase and lactate dehydrogenase deficiency.

In myopathies due to *fatty acid transport and oxidation defects* (Di Donato, 1994; Roe & Coates, 1995; Brumback et al., 1992), hepatic synthesis of ketone bodies and the energy production at rest and during muscular contraction are impaired. Clinical conditions vary according to onset and severity. The main clinical features are: intolerance to prolonged exercise and paroxysmal myoglobinuria (both of which are favoured by fasting, cold and infections); intolerance to fasting, with recurrent episodes of hypoketotic hypoglycaemia, sometimes with transitory neurological disorders; lipid storage myopathy (LSM), cardiomyopathy, Reye's syndrome, sudden infant death syndrome (SIDS), and congenital anomalies with polycystic kidney. These myopathies can be subdivided into two groups:

defects of the carnitine cycle including defects of carnitine transporter, carnitine palmitoyltransferase (CPT) I and II and carnitine-acylcarnitine translocase;

defects of beta-oxidation, including both isolated defects of short-chain acyl-CoA dehydrogenase (SCAD), medium-chain acyl-CoA dehydrogenase (MCAD), long-chain acyl-CoA dehydrogenase (LCAD), very long-chain acyl-CoA dehydrogenase, 3-OH acyl-CoA dehydrogenase (HAD) and multiple acyl-CoA dehydrogenase deficiency (MADD) or glutaric aciduria type II, including the riboflavin-responsive form. Dicarboxylic aciduria and hypoketonaemia are generally the markers of these disorders.

Mitochondrial diseases now have an 'expanding clinical spectrum' stemming from the exponential development of knowledge in this field (De Vivo, 1993). According to the genetic classification proposed by De Vivo, these are subdivideable into:

nuclear DNA defects, inherited through the mendelian autosomal recessive mechanism, including defects of ß-oxidation (usually considered independently), defects of the pyruvate dehydrogenase complex and respiratory chain defects;

mitochondrial DNA (mtDNA) defects, due to sporadic large-scale rearrangements and maternally inherited point mutations affecting structural and synthetic genes;

intergenomic signalling defects, including autosomal dominant multiple mtDNA deletions and autosomal recessive mtDNA depletion.

Generally, their clinical features are very heterogeneous (De Vivo, 1993; Morgan-Hughes, 1994; Dubowitz, 1995; Saudubray & Charpentier, 1995): onset at any age; a clinical picture ranging from exercise intolerance or recurrent myoglobinuria to severe forms and from isolated myopathy to multisystemic forms; the presence of transitory, recurrent, slowly progressive, or rapidly lethal forms. The morphological hallmark of mtDNA lesions affecting intramitochondrial protein synthesis is the presence of ragged-red fibres (RRF), seen with the modified Gomori trichrome stain and related to the subsarcolemmal proliferation of mitochondria.

An *anomaly of purine metabolism* (Sabina & Holmes, 1995; Brumback et al., 1992), the myoadenylate deaminase deficiency, causes cramps and myoglobinuria. Soft muscles and benign congenital hypotonia can be associated, but progressive myopathy rarely occurs. This deficiency may be inherited as an autosomal recessive trait.

Clinical approach

The *clinical approach* is based on the following parameters: family history, age at onset, muscular findings, triggering factors, and muscular symptoms either isolated or associated with heart, liver, CNS and other organ involvement.

Laboratory examinations include preliminary tests such as assays of muscular and hepatic enzymes, lactate, pyruvate, ketone bodies, ammonia, and triglycerides, followed by more specific investigations such as lactate/pyruvate ratio before and after meals, organic aciduria and assay of free and esterified carnitine.

Further data are obtained by electrophysiological studies, as described below. In histochemical and histoenzymatic assays, the muscular biopsy can show lipid and glycogen storage, RRF, or oxidative reaction anomalies and can demonstrate myophosphorylase, phosphofructokinase, cytochrome c oxidase and myoadenylate deaminase deficiency. Finally, in several diseases, enzyme assay and additional genetic studies can be performed. A correct clinical approach enables a simplified diagnostic protocol and an acceptable cost–benefit ratio.

Family history can be an important clue leading to diagnosis. Maternal, dominant and X-linked inheritance could suggest mtDNA point mutations, multiple mtDNA deletions, and GSD type IX, respectively (Di Mauro & Tsujino, 1994; De Vivo, 1993; Morgan-Hughes, 1994).

Age at onset is a significant aspect, given that many disorders are age-related (Saudubray & Charpentier, 1995).

A few defects, occurring in the foetal period, lead to congenital anomalies, namely MADD, CPT II deficiency and pyruvate defects. Many severe neonatal forms can be ascribed to fatty acid oxidation, respiratory chain and pyruvate defects. Pompe's disease occurs in the first months of life and quickly worsens. At other ages, a wide spectrum of disorders can occur; in adolescence, deficiencies related to exercise intolerance with myoglobinuria are particularly frequent.

Muscular findings can be *aspecific* and have the same pattern as other myopathies, such as severe or benign congenital hypotonia, progressive myopathies differing according to the degree and localization of muscular weakness, and asymptomatic creatine kinase (CK) increase.

By contrast, some features, such as *exercise* or *fasting intolerance* and *acute rhabdomyolysis*, suggest a metabolic ætiology. Further insight into this matter requires more information on the mechanisms underlying normal muscle metabolism (Brumback *et al.*, 1992; Di Mauro & Tsujino, 1994; Saudubray & Charpentier, 1995; Tonin *et al.*, 1990).

In the resting state, the muscle is dependent on fatty acid oxidation. During moderate exercise, blood glucose is also utilized. During short and intense exercise, ATP production also requires muscular glycogen, whereas during intense and prolonged exercise, muscular lipids are utilized. After meals, the muscle uses mainly glucides and, after prolonged fasting, employs lipids and ketone bodies.

Short and intense exercise intolerance causes painful contractures. The disappearance of painful contractures after a short rest and the subsequent possibility of prolonging the exercise ('second wind' phenomenon) can occur, probably reflecting a switch from carbohydrate to fatty acid utilization. In late childhood and adolescence, this intolerance is typically due to glycogenolysis or glycolysis deficiency, mainly GSD type V or McArdle's disease.

Mild or moderate prolonged exercise intolerance, especially during fasting, cold or infections, causes muscle pain, weakness and stiffness, but no severe exercise-induced contractures. It occurs in adolescents rather than in children and is mainly due to CPT II deficiency.

A less characteristic exercise intolerance with weakness has been described in myoadenylate deaminase, respiratory chain and fatty acid oxidation deficiencies (Saudubray & Charpentier, 1995).

In *acute rhabdomyolysis* (Brumback et al., 1992), the breakdown of skeletal muscle cells causes the release of their contents into the circulation, with high serum creatine phosphokinase levels, hyperkalaemia, hyperphosphatemia and myoglobinuria. Among metabolic disorders, CPT deficiency may play a principal role in the above-mentioned diseases determining exercise intolerance (Tonin et al., 1990).

The *forearm ischaemic exercise test* is the classic test for identifying patients with defects of muscle energy metabolism. Ischaemia is achieved by inflating the blood pressure cuff to above systolic blood pressure and the patient is asked to squeeze a dynamometer or a partially inflated roll cuff of another blood-pressure apparatus 40 times per min or up to exhaustion or contracture. Blood is sampled from the ischaemic forearm before the exercise and at 1, 3, 5, 10 and 20 min to determine lactate and ammonia. If possible, CK should be assayed at rest and after 4, 8, 12 and 24 h. Urine is collected before and after the exercise to detect myoglobinuria. In normal individuals, lactate shows a three- to fivefold rise over the resting level in the first 2–3 min, returning to the pre-exercise level in 20 min; ammonia levels show a two- to threefold increase over the resting level. If this does not occur, the test is not satisfactory and must be repeated. Patients with myophosphorylase deficiency are able to exercise for approximately 1 min before the onset of severe painful muscle contraction. Lactate levels do not increase significantly, whereas ammonia shows a three- to fivefold increase over the resting levels. Serum CK levels are elevated and hyperuricaemia and myoglobinuria may be observed. In GSD type III, an intermediate increase with respect to normal range indicates the presence of debrancher enzyme deficiency also in the muscle. The lack of increase in ammonia associated with normal lactate rise suggests a myoadenylate deaminase deficiency, even if false positives are not rare. An excessive lactate increase points to a mitochondrial disease.

Electrophysiological examinations provide some further information. In fact, some tests are available to detect GSD types V or VII (Kimura, 1984). During the ischaemic exercise test, the simultaneous EMG recording of finger deep-flexor muscles shows electrical silence in severely contracted muscles, lasting briefly after the end of ischaemia, whereas in ordinary cramps or spasms abundant discharges of motor unit potentials are recorded. The repetitive stimulation above threshold (at 18/s) of the median nerve induces a severe cramp in thenar eminence muscles and a rapid amplitude decrement of compound muscle action potential. In infancy or childhood, however, exercise intolerance is not usually observed and is, moreover, difficult to detect.

By contrast, a metabolic disease can be suspected in the presence of *abnormal fatiguability* and *fluctuating muscular weakness*, depending on fasting and motor activity or occurring intercurrent illness.

At times, 'myasthenic-like' aspects can be observed as well. In particular, they are often revealed in respiratory chain and ß-oxidation defects.

The problem of *provocation tests* then arises. The exercise test can be performed only if adapted to the very young patient and often has to be supplemented by the mother's active collaboration. Depending on age and weakness, the child is invited to climb stairs or to walk on a flat surface for as long as possible.

In the fasting test, prolonged fasting should be avoided as it might trigger acute metabolic distress, but moderate fasting, e.g. necessary for an anaesthetic procedure, can be utilized.

Due to the wider ætiological spectrum in infancy and childhood, the assay of pyruvate, glycaemia, ketone bodies and amino acids is also required, but should be performed only twice, before and after the test.

Muscular symptoms can be *isolated or associated with extramuscular involvement*. The latter can appear before, during or after muscular skeletal symptoms, and is mainly chronic and progressive. It is likely to be related to the different tissue-specific subunits and can provide information useful in establishing the diagnostic procedures to adopt.

In infancy and childhood, metabolic myopathies often cause *cardiomyopathies* (CMP), either hypertrophic or dilated, or both in sequence. According to Saudubray & Charpentier (1995), a CMP can be a predominant or revealing symptom, an isolated finding or part of a known clinical picture. In the first case, hypotonia and failure to thrive are frequently observed.

In mitochondrial respiratory-chain diseases, heart involvement is not an unexpected finding, since myocardial cells are very rich in mitochondria and depend considerably on aerobic metabolism. This accounts for the observation of heart involvement in 10 per cent of mitochondrial diseases, and of mitochondrial ætiology in 20 per cent of nonobstructive dilated myocardiopathies in the first year of life. The presence of ketoacidosis and hyperlactacidaemia in a subject with psychomotor retardation facilitates the diagnosis. SIDS can also occur. The deficiencies most frequently observed involve complexes I, II and IV of the respiratory chain.

A CMP with massive widespread storage is typically due to Pompe's disease (Engel & Hirschhorn, 1994; Dubowitz, 1995). Signs of heart failure can already be observed in the first months and even in the first weeks of life. They are rapidly followed (but sometimes preceded) by muscular hypotonia. A weak cry, facial weakness, astonished look, and macroglossia are tell-tale signs. CK is increased and the peripheral smear shows vacuolated lymphocytes. The ECG shows a short PR interval, high QRS voltage and left ventricular hypertrophy. The EMG, usually demonstrating aspecific myopathic signs, in Pompe's disease shows a diagnostic pattern (Kimura, 1984), characterized by the association of myopathic signs and abnormal spontaneous activity: increased insertion activity, diffuse fibrillation, positive sharp potentials, and the particular finding of bizarre high-frequency discharges differing from true myotonic discharges in the absence of decrement and of clinical myotonia. In our experience, its identification has been very useful in the CMP diagnostic protocol (Veneselli, 1991).

In the anomalies of fatty acid oxidation (Di Donato, 1994; Saudubray & Charpentier, 1995), the heart, together with skeletal muscle and liver, is a target organ, since fatty acids and ketone bodies are its main energy sources. In infancy and childhood, muscular involvement can be misdiagnosed and identified with hypotonia related to heart failure. The occurrence of hypoketotic hypoglycaemia, however, leads to its diagnosis. The metabolic anomalies more frequently detected are carnitine cycle defects (but not CPT I), LCAD and MAD deficiency. In particular, a toxic role of long-chain acyl-CoA in mitochondrial phosphorylation has been hypothesized.

In infancy and childhood, an isolated CMP is mainly related to respiratory chain defects, but a deficiency of phosphorylase b kinase is possible. By contrast, in late childhood, CMP is usually part of a more extensive clinical involvement: for instance, hepatomegaly with hypoglycaemia in GSD type III and liver failure with cirrhosis in GSD type IV.

Heartbeat disorders, including complete heart block, can be observed in several diseases, mainly in the acute forms of fatty acid oxidation defects in newborns and infants (appearing as SIDS) (Saudubray & Charpentier, 1995). In late childhood, heart block occurs in Kearns–Sayre syndrome (KSS) (De Vivo, 1993).

A metabolic myopathy with significant *liver dysfunction* occurs in some conditions (Di Mauro, 1994; Di Donato, 1994; Roe & Coates, 1995; Zierz, 1994; Saudubray & Charpentier, 1995). Liver involvement is the predominant sign in GSD types III and IV. In early childhood, a permanent hepatomegaly suggests the presence of GSD type IV, when the clinical picture is severe, with cirrhosis, splenomegaly, and failure to thrive. On the contrary, a moderate clinical picture with marked hepatomegaly and hypoglycaemic episodes suggests GSD type III. According to the literature and in our experience (Di Mauro & Tsujino, 1994; Dubowitz, 1995; Veneselli, 1991), a long follow-up of these patients is very important, since the natural history of GSD type III is characterized by a progressive disappearance of liver dysfunction with a correct diet, but also by the late appearance of myopathy, CMP and peripheral neuropathy. In order to prevent or delay the late-onset symptoms, continuation of the diet after puberal development is compulsory.

A wide range of liver dysfunctions occurs in lipidic and mitochondrial disorders, including a marked increase in transaminases, episodes of hypoglycaemia, liver steatosis, and acute failure. This is more evident in fatty acid oxidation defects, where liver dysfunction is usually the major problem and can lead to cirrhosis (Di Donato, 1994; Roe & Coates, 1995; Saudubray & Charpentier, 1995).

Acute liver disease is the most significant event in *Reye's syndrome* and Reye-like disorders (Green & Hall, 1992; Saudubray & Charpentier, 1995).

Reye's syndrome is an acute non-inflammatory encephalopathy of undefined ætiopathogenesis, related to severe liver dysfunction. After a common infection, acute hepatocellular failure with steatosis is rapidly followed by lethargy, convulsions, coma, cerebral oedema, and severe hyperthermia; myopathy, cardiomyopathy and signs of other organ involvement, mainly of the kidneys, are often observed. According to the British Reye's Syndrome Surveillance Scheme (BRSSS) (Green & Hall, 1992), the syndrome is defined as an unexplained non-inflammatory encephalopathy, occurring in children under 16 years, and associated with one or more of the following: (a) serum hepatic transaminase increased ≥ 3 times over the normal limit; (b) plasma ammonia concentration increased ≥ 3 times over the normal limit; (c) characteristic fatty infiltration of the liver.

Over the last decade in the UK, inherited metabolic disorders have accounted for over 40 per cent of cases of Reye-like syndrome (10 per cent reported as Reye's syndrome itself), with a prevalence of MCAD defects (Green & Hall, 1992). This prevalence is confirmed in a similar French series (Saudubray & Charpentier, 1995).

According to the BRSSS, an inherited metabolic disorder should be suspected in any child presenting at least one of the following characteristics: age < 3 years; a past history of encephalopathic episodes; vomiting during viral infections, an unexplained failure to thrive, neurodevelopmental disorders, and near-miss SIDS; a family history of RS, SIDS and unexplained encephalopathy; no history of viral prodromes clearly separated from the onset of encephalopathy.

The involvement of both the CNS and muscle, i.e. *encephalomyopathies*, is uniquely interesting from the point of view of developmental neurology. Whereas the encephalomyopathies observed in congenital, progressive and myotonic muscular dystrophies have well-known and stereotyped neurological patterns, metabolic encephalomyopathies present extremely heterogeneous conditions.

Encephalomyopathies can also be observed in glycogenoses (Di Mauro & Tsujino, 1994). Cerebral involvement is possible in advanced stages of classical GSD types II and IV and in some particular forms such as lactic dehydrogenase deficiency with mental retardation, atypical cases of GSD types V and VII, 'cardiomyopathy, mental retardation, autophagic vacuolar myopathy' with glycogen storage but unknown biochemical defect.

In fatty acid oxidation defects (Di Donato, 1994; Roe & Coates, 1995; Saudubray & Charpentier, 1995), various clinical phenotypes are observed, including congenital anomalies, neonatal neurological distress due to 'intoxication' or 'energy deficiency', intermittent late-onset acute neurological presentations with hepatic signs, Reye's syndrome and SIDS; psychomotor delay, mental retardation and sometimes seizures are also observed (Saudubray & Charpentier, 1995).

A peculiar condition is the Bannayan–Riley–Ruvalcaba syndrome with megalencephaly, mental retardation, and lipid storage myopathy. LCAD deficiency has been recently identified (Fryburg *et al.*, 1994).

Mitochondrial diseases (De Vivo, 1993; Morgan-Hughes, 1994; Dubowitz, 1995; Saudubray & Charpentier, 1995) present a very wide spectrum of neurological phenotypes. On the basis of the main clinical findings reported in the literature, these diseases should be suspected when any of the following features are associated: mental deterioration, epilepsy, myoclonus, ataxia, peripheral neuropathy, stroke-like episodes, neurosensorial deafness, pigmentary retinopathy, CMP, growth deficiency, cutaneous anomalies, diabetes, hypoparathyroidism, pancreatic insufficiency, chronic diarrhoea, tubulopathy, vitamin-resistant rickets, pancytopenia, or macrocytic anaemia.

The diagnostic approach is quite easy in the case of well-known syndromes. KSS, included in the group of mtDNA large-scale rearrangements, is characterized by the invariant triad of clinical symptoms including childhood onset, progressive ophthalmoparesis and pigmentary retinopathy, together with cerebellar syndrome, elevation of the CSF protein, and propensity to complete heart block. The syndromes related to mtDNA point mutations are mitochondrial encephalomyopathy with lactic acidosis and stroke-like episodes (MELAS) and myoclonus epilepsy and RRF (MERRF). Progressive external ophthalmoplegias (PEO), related to different mtDNA defects, provide another suggestive phenotype. Electrophysiological and neuroradiological examinations are particularly useful in this group of disorders.

An extensive neurophysiological evaluation (EEG, EMG, NCV, ABR, SEP, VEP, ERG) allows the identification of multiple, even subclinical, dysfunctions, such as signs of brainstem dysfunction, neurosensorial hearing loss and retinal degeneration. At times, patterns suggestive of MELAS and MERRF can be detected.

Neuroimaging can reveal aspecific findings including white matter anomalies and/or cortico-subcortical atrophy, but also more significant features, such as basal ganglia abnormalities, in a few forms, or even diagnostic findings such as multifocal laminar cortical patterns in MELAS (Leutner et al., 1994; Matthews et al., 1991).

Conclusions

The clinical approach to metabolic myopathies requires diagnostic algorithms to identify inherited disorders. It includes an accurate evaluation of all the parameters in a thorough and integrated manner. As in any scheme, it is difficult to satisfy the need to identify categories of practical usefulness and, at the same time, to take into account deranging conditions.

The specific detection of enzyme deficiency or of genetic markers in some diseases is relatively simple, for instance acid maltase assay on circulating leukocytes, but more often it demands the multidisciplinary collaboration of advanced specialized centres.

The diagnostic target is important. A therapeutic approach is possible in some diseases: for instance, it can prevent or delay the onset of myopathy in GSD type III, reduce the severity of rhabdomyolytic episodes and resolve carnitine- and riboflavin-responsive MAD deficiencies. Moreover, prenatal diagnosis can be performed in any form with a known enzyme deficiency or identified genetic marker. The journal *Neuromuscular Disorders* provides useful updates on the gene location of myopathies and the gene mutations of mitochondrial myopathies.

References

Brumback, R.A., Feeback, D.L. & Leech, R.W. (1992): Rhabdomyolysis in childhood. A primer on normal muscle function and selected metabolic myopathies characterized by disordered energy production. *Pediatr. Clin. North Am.* **39**, 821–858.

De Vivo, D.C. (1993): The expanding clinical spectrum of mitochondrial diseases. *Brain Dev.* **15**, 1–22.

Di Donato, S. (1994): Disorders of lipid metabolism affecting skeletal muscle: carnitine deficiency syndromes, defects in the catabolic pathway, and Chanarin disease. In: *Myology*, eds. A.G. Engel & C. Franzini-Armstrong, pp. 1587–1609. New York: McGraw-Hill.

DiMauro, S. & Tsujino, S. (1994): Nonlysosomal glycogenoses. In: *Myology*, eds. A.G. Engel & C. Franzini-Armstrong, pp. 1554–1576. New York: McGraw-Hill.

Dubowitz, V. (1995): *Muscle disorders in childhood.* London: W.B. Saunders Co.

Engel, A.G. & Hirschhorn, R. (1994): Acid maltase deficiency. In: *Myology*, eds. A.G. Engel & C. Franzini-Armstrong, pp. 1533–1553. New York: McGraw-Hill.

Fryburg, J.S., Pelegano, J.P., Bennett, M.J. & Bebin, E.M. (1994): Long-chain 3-hydroxyacyl-Coenzyme: A dehydrogenase (L-CHAD) deficiency in a patient with the Bannayan-Riley-Ruvalcaba syndrome. *Am. J. Med. Genet.* **52,** 97–102.

Green, A. & Hall, S.M. (1992): Investigation of metabolic disorders resembling Reye's syndrome. *Arch. Dis. Child.* **67,** 1313–1317.

Kimura, J. (1984): *Electrodiagnosis in diseases of nerve and muscle: principles and practice.* Philadelphia: F.A. Davis Co.

Leutner, C., Layer, G., Zierz, S., Solymosi, L., Dewes, W. & Reiser, M. (1994): Cerebral MR in ophthalmoplegia plus. *Am. J. Neuroradiol.* **15,** 681–687.

Matthews, P.M., Phil, D., Tampieri, D., Berkovic, S.F., Andermann, F., Silver, K., Chityat, D. & Arnold, D.L. (1991): Magnetic resonance imaging shows specific abnormalities in the MELAS syndrome. *Neurology* **41,** 1043–1046.

Morgan-Hughes J.A. (1994): Mitochondrial diseases. In: *Myology*, eds. A.G. Engel & C. Franzini-Armstrong, pp. 1610–1660. New York: McGraw-Hill.

Roe, C.R. and Coates, P.M. (1995): Mitochondrial fatty acid oxidation disorders. In: *The metabolic and molecular bases of inherited disease*, eds. C.R. Scriver, A.L. Beaudet, W.S. Sly & D. Valle, p. 1501. New York: McGraw-Hill.

Sabina, R.L. & Holmes E.W. (1995): Myoadenylate deaminase deficiency. In: *The metabolic and molecular bases of inherited disease*, eds. C.R. Scriver, A.L. Beaudet, W.S. Sly. & D. Valle, pp. 1769–1780. New York: McGraw-Hill.

Saudubray, J.M. & Charpentier, C. (1995): Clinical phenotypes: diagnosis/algorithms. In: *The metabolic and molecular bases of inherited disease*, eds. C.R. Scriver, A.L. Beaudet, W.S. Sly. & D. Valle, pp. 327–400. New York: McGraw-Hill.

Tonin, P., Lewis, P., Servidei, S. & Di Mauro, S. (1990): Metabolic causes of myoglobinuria. *Ann. Neurol.* **27,** 181–185.

Veneselli, E. (1991): Aspetti elettromiografici delle miopatie metaboliche. *Minerva Pediatr.* **43,** 107–110.

Zierz S. (1994): Carnitine palmitoyltransferase deficiency. In: *Myology,* eds. A.G. Engel & C. Franzini-Armstrong, pp. 1577–1586. New York: McGraw-Hill.

Chapter 2

Clinical heterogeneity of the respiratory chain defects

Enrico Bertini,[1] Serenella Servidei,[2] Enzo Ricci,[2] Gabriella Silvestri,[2] Carlo Dionisi Vici,[1] Carlo Piantadosi[1] and Pietro Tonali[1]

[1]*Neurophysiological Service, Bambino Gesù Hospital, Piazza S. Onofrio 4, 00165 Rome;*
[2]*Neurological Institute, Catholic University, Largo Gemelli, 00168 Rome, Italy*

Summary

Patients affected by mitochondrial (mt) respiratory chain defects (RCD) show remarkable clinical heterogeneity. Clinically these disorders usually affect muscles either alone or in combination with other systems, most often the brain (encephalomyopathies).

The respiratory chain contains five functional units or complexes that are localized in the inner mitochondrial membrane. Unlike the other metabolic pathways present in the mitochondria, respiratory chain functional units are under the control of two genomes: the nuclear DNA (nDNA) and the mitochondrial genome (mtDNA). Therefore, RCD may be caused by mutations of nDNA, mtDNA or defects that involve intergenomic communication.

Defects of nDNA encoded subunits biochemically affect the activity of single complexes and can cause tissue-specific or generalized enzyme deficiencies. This may explain the variable tissue involvement in some mendelian inherited respiratory chain defects.

mtDNA derives entirely from the maternal oocyte; each mitochondrion contains up to 10 mtDNAs and each cell contains thousands of mt genomes. Pathogenetic mtDNA mutations are by definition generalized, but the phenotypic involvement of each tissue will depend on the relative proportion of mutant mtDNA in that tissue (heteroplasmy) and on its relative dependence on oxidative phosphorylation (threshold effect). Biochemical defects may be partial and sometimes undetectable by routine methods.

Defects of intergenomic communication are due to primary mutations in nDNA and cause secondary mtDNA lesions (multiple deletions or mtDNA depletion).

After clinical suspicion, extensive investigations must be performed in order to obtain a correct diagnosis of RCD. Preliminary selection of patients by metabolic examination of body fluids, particularly measurement of serum lactate/pyruvate and acetoacetate/3-OH-butyrate ratio as well as CSF lactate, is crucial. *In vivo* function tests such as brain proton MR spectroscopy and exercise tolerance test with an ergometer may increase evidence of a mt RCD. Primary RCD must be proven by morphological, genetic and biochemical criteria.

Most of mt proteins are encoded by nDNA and are imported from the cytoplasm into the mitochondria by mechanisms that are under the control of the nDNA. Several nDNA encoded factors also control mtDNA replication, transcription and translation. Mitochondrial disorders due to nDNA mutations are transmitted as mendelian traits and provoke (1) alterations of mt proteins, (2) alterations of mt protein importation and (3) alterations in intergenomic communication. The first group of disorders can be further classified biochemically (Di Mauro, 1993): (a) defects of substrate transport, (b) defects of substrate utilization, (c) defects of Krebs cycle, (d) defects of oxidation/phosphorylation coupling, and (e) defects of respiratory chain (RCD). We will limit our review to the increasingly large subject of RCD, describing the main clinical features and the diagnostic methodology.

These disorders usually affect muscles either alone or in combination with other systems, most often brain (encephalomyopathies) and heart. RCD may result from a molecular defect involving mitochondrial mtDNA or nDNA. The respiratory chain contains five functional units or complexes that are localized in the inner mitochondrial membrane. Unlike the other metabolic pathways present in the mitochondria, respiratory chain functional units are influenced by the nDNA as well as the mtDNA. The five complexes contain approximately 70 polypeptides, 13 of which are encoded by mtDNA. In addition, mtDNA contains 24 genes for its own protein synthesis which include two ribosomal RNAs and 22 transfer RNAs (tRNAs).

The concepts of heteroplasmy, replicative mitotic segregation and threshold effect have provided the theoretical background for the variable phenotypic expression in the same kindred of maternally transmitted human diseases due to mtDNA mutations (see Di Mauro & Moraes, 1993; Wallace & Lott, 1993; De Vivo, 1993 for additional reading). Pathogenetic mutations of mtDNA are by definition generalized, but the phenotypic involvement of each tissue will depend on the relative proportion of mutant mtDNA in that tissue (heteroplasmy) and on its relative dependence on oxidative phosphorylation (threshold effect). Biochemical defects are partial and sometimes difficult to detect by routine methods.

The notion of tissue-specific mitochondrial nuclear-encoded subunits could give the basis to explain the variable tissue involvement in some mendelian inherited RCD. Mutations of nDNA may affect the activity of single complexes or involve factors for intergenomic communication, such as in autosomal dominant progressive external ophthalmoplegia (PEO) with multiple deletions or in mtDNA depletion, causing multiple and partial biochemical complex defects. This subject has been particularly studied in infantile complex IV or cytochrome oxidase (COX) disorders with defects in nDNA-encoded subunits in which tissue specific and generalized forms of COX deficiency have been reported. However, although molecular probes for all the nDNA-encoded COX subunits are available, molecular defects causing mendelian inherited disorders are still unknown (Di Mauro et al., 1993).

In the diagnosis of mitochondrial encephalomyopathies, after clinical suspicion, extensive morphological, biochemical and genetical investigations may be necessary to obtain a correct assessment. It is therefore important to carry out a preliminary selection of patients to find a biochemical marker suggesting impairment of oxidative phosphorylation. Metabolic examination of body fluids, particularly measurement of the ratios of serum lactate/pyruvate (L/P) and acetoacetate/3-OH-butyrate (HB/AA) during fed and fasting states, is of crucial importance to demonstrate primary lactic acidosis (Trijbels et al., 1988; Bonnefont et al., 1990; Vassault et al., 1991). Hyperlactacidaemia is a near constant finding in RCD but can be moderate (2–3 mmol/l). In such situations, CSF lactate and blood lactate measurements after a glucose load test could be useful. The L/P ratio is high and is frequently associated with postprandial, paradoxical hyperchetonaemia and a high 3-HOB/AA ratio (Vassault et al., 1991). Measurement of serum carnitine and serum and urinary amino acids may also be an additional tool to outline characteristic disorders (Perry et al., 1989) or Fanconi syndrome. Urinary lactate by gas chromatography and mass spectroscopy (GC/MS) is also very useful; GC/MS can detect additional organic acids in RCD, such as Krebs cycle precursors or 3-methylglutaconic aciduria (Jakobs et al., 1991; Gibson et al., 1992; Bennett et al., 1993). Urinary organic acids may be peculiar to specific syndromes like ethylmalonic aciduria-acrocyanosis-relapsing petechiae-chronic diarrhoea-spasticity-mental retardation (Burlina et al., 1994) or 3-methylglutaconic aciduria-mitochondrial myopathy and cardiopathy-multiple respiratory chain defects including ATPase (Holme et al., 1992), 3-methylglutaconic aciduria and X-linked cardiomyopathy (Kelley et al., 1991) and Leigh syndrome with biotinidase deficiency (Baumgartner et al., 1989). In vivo function tests such as brain magnetic resonance spectroscopy (MRS) are able to measure brain lactate by ^{1}H-MRS (Detre et al., 1991; Tzika et al., 1994; Mathews et al., 1994) or muscle and brain energy metabolism by ^{31}P-MRS (Lodi et al., 1994), particularly in instances where blood lactate may not be elevated. In co-operative patients, venous blood lactate can also be measured after a sub-anaerobic threshold test by an ergometer and is useful to identify patients with abnormalities of muscle energy metabolism (Nashef & Lane, 1989). Primary RCD must be proven by morphological, genetic and biochemical criteria. Biochemical examination is generally performed in fresh or frozen muscle biopsies and the functioning of the electron transport chain can be established by measuring the oxidation rates of several mitochondrial substrates. The functional capacity of mitochondrial oxidative phosphorylation can also be studied in cultured fibroblasts (Wanders et al., 1993) and screening methods can be applied using glucose-incubated fibroblasts and measuring lactate to pyruvate ratios (Robinson et al., 1990) or measuring survival of fibroblasts in culture medium with galactose (Robinson et al., 1992).

Morphological criteria

Muscle biopsy is a very important step in the diagnosis of mitochondrial myopathies and encephalomyopathies. It should be performed, if possible, after clinical symptoms and screening methods have given strong evidence that we are dealing with a disorder of oxydative phosphorylation.

More than 30 years after their description (Engel & Cunningham, 1963), the ragged-red fibres (RRF), shown in Fig. 1A and B, caused by segmental accumulation of mitochondria, are still considered a morphological hallmark of many mitochondrial encephalomyopathies (Rowland et al., 1991). RRF have been almost invariably documented in disorders causing impaired mtDNA protein synthesis (large scale mtDNA deletions, mtDNA point mutations of genes encoding for tRNAs and mtDNA depletion). On the other hand mitochondrial encephalomyopathies due to nDNA defects (Leigh syndrome) or due to mtDNA point mutations of structural genes – Leber hereditary optic neuropathy(LHON) and neutrogenic atrophy, ataxia, retinitis pigmentosa (NARP) – do not show RRF. Histochemical reaction for succinate dehydrogenase (SDH) is a very sensitive method of detecting RRF (Fig. 1A); the histochemical reaction for COX shows that RRF are frequently COX negative (see Fig. 1A and B for comments)

Clinical, genetic and biochemical classification in RCD

A rational classification of RCD is based on genetic criteria and distinguishes three major categories: (1) defects in mtDNA; (2) defects in intergenomic communication; (3) defects in nDNA (Di Mauro, 1993). Following this classification we will briefly review the most important clinical syndromes.

I. Clinical syndromes associated with defects of mtDNA

Disorders due to mtDNA point mutations are maternally inherited while disorders due to large-scale mtDNA deletions are generally sporadic. Defects of mtDNA may be classified by clinical syndromes or by genetic lesions. However, there is frequently no full phenotype–genotype correlation: the same syndrome can be caused by different mtDNA defects and conversely, the same mutation can cause different clinical syndromes (Di Mauro & Moraes, 1993). New clinical syndromes and genetical mtDNA mutations are continuously updated in *Neuromuscular Disorders* (by Servidei).

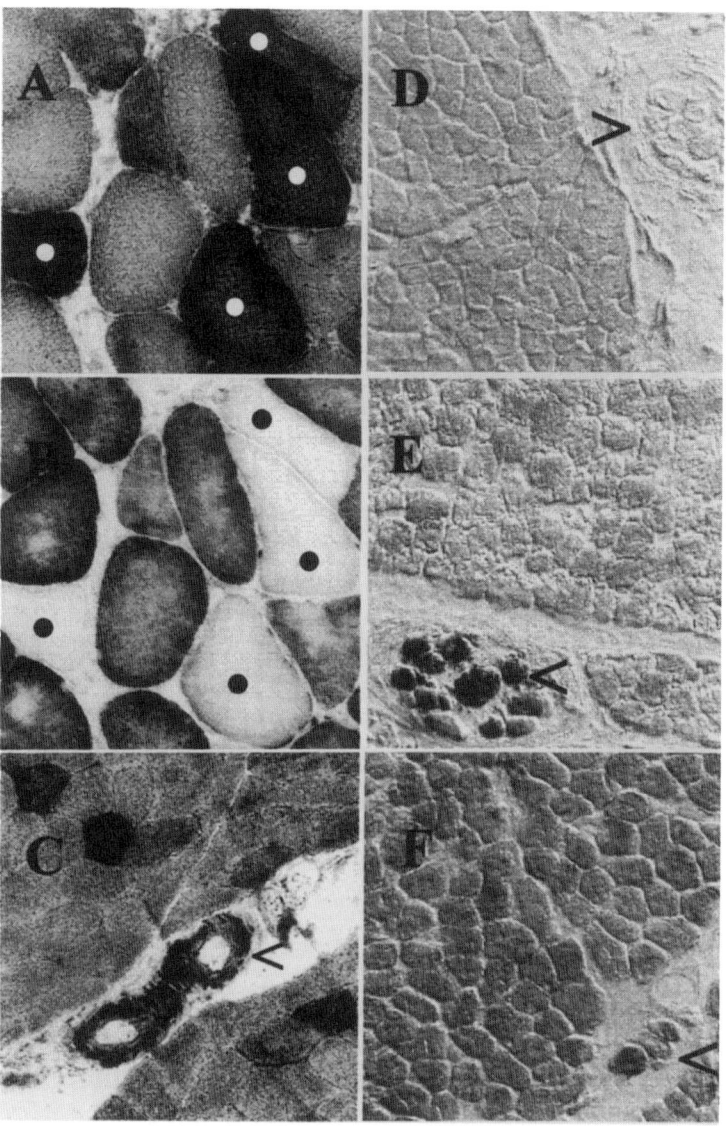

*Fig. 1. Morphological findings in muscle of some mitochondrial encephalomyopathies. (**A** and **B**) adult patient with PEO and mtDNA large-scale deletion; serial cryostat sections are stained for SDH (A) and COX (B). RRF (dotted on SDH) are COX negative indicating the association of mitochondrial proliferation and a biochemical RCD. (**C**) adult patient with MELAS mutation at the nt3243. Section is stained for SDH and shows strongly succinate dehydrogenase-reactive blood vessel walls (open arrow head). (**D**) child with Leigh disease and COX deficiency; both intrafusal (open arrow head) and extrafusal muscle fibres are COX deficient. (**E**) child with fatal infantile COX deficiency; COX activity is deficient only in extrafusal fibres and normal in intrafusal fibres (open arrow head) suggesting tissue-specific COX deficiency. (**F**) 10-month-old child with normal COX staining (control). Sections of D, E, F were attached and stained for COX in the same slide.*

Mitochondrial encephalopathy, lactic acidosis, stroke-like episodes (MELAS)

This syndrome is characterized by the association of: (1) mitochondrial encephalopathy (particularly seizures and dementia), (2) lactic acidosis or RRF and (3) stroke-like episodes before the age of 40 years. In a large review of 69 cases with MELAS syndrome, additional important clinical features were found to be normal early development, recurrent headaches or recurrent vomiting (Hirano et al., 1992). Sometimes there are overlap symptoms between MELAS and myoclonic epilepsy ragged-red fibres (MERRF) or Kearns–Sayre syndrome (KSS) but in these cases associated syndromes do not express the full symptoms. Morphologically the presence of RRF in the muscle biopsy are important for diagnosis but mitochondrial proliferation is frequently seen in vessels as strongly succinate dehydrogenase-reactive vessel walls (Fig. 1C) (Hasegawa et al., 1991). In MELAS, DNA mutations generally involve the tRNA $^{Leu(UUR)}$ gene. The most common mutation (about 80–90 per cent of patients) is at nt3243 (A→G) which was first described by Goto et al. (1990). Biochemical abnormalities of respiratory chain may be absent in about 20 per cent of cases (Hirano & Pavlakis, 1994). MELAS is not the only clinical expression of the 3243 mutation or other tRNA $^{Leu(UUR)}$ mutations; about one-third of patients with PEO and RRF, but without mtDNA deletion, have the 3243 mutation (Moraes et al., 1993). Moreover, the same mutation at nt3243 has been described in diabetes/deafness syndrome (Van den Ouweland et al., 1994) and in progressive dystonia (Johns et al., 1994) For the other mutations of the tRNA $^{Leu(UUR)}$ see *Neuromuscular Disorders*.

Myoclonic epilepsy, ragged-red fibres (MERRF)

This syndrome was first described by Fukuhara et al. in 1980. They reviewed the literature and suggested that this disorder was a specific entity and had similarities with Friedreich's ataxia and the Ramsey Hunt syndrome. In this disorder the most common symptoms are ataxia, exercise intolerance, generalized convulsions, myoclonus, dementia, hearing loss, and neuropathy (Pavlakis et al., 1988). A muscle biopsy shows fibres with mitochondrial proliferation (RRF) and COX deficient fibres. The most common mutation is at nt 8344 (A→G) in the tRNA^{Lys} gene (Shoffner et al., 1990). Other rare phenotypes associated with this mutation include Leigh syndrome, isolated proximal myopathy (Silvestri et al., 1993) and Ekbom syndrome: lipomas, ataxia and neuropathy (Calabresi et al., 1994). The same MERRF syndrome (Silvestri et al., 1992) and an overlap MERRF/MELAS syndrome (Zeviani et al., 1993) have been associated with another mutation at the nt8356 (T→C).

Progressive external ophthalmoplegia (PEO), Kearns–Sayre syndrome (KSS), Pearson syndrome and other syndromes with large scale mtDNA rearrangements

KSS was described in 1958 (Kearns & Sayre, 1958), long before the description of the first mtDNA deletion by Holt et al. (1988). It is characterized by the association of three symptoms: (1) onset before 20 years of age; (2) PEO; (3) pigmentary retinopathy plus at least one of the following: heart block, cerebellar ataxia, or increased protein concentration in the cerebrospinal fluid (Di Mauro, 1993). Southern blot analysis generally shows single, large-scale deletions in most cases and insertions/duplications in a few (Poulton et al., 1989). Some cases with large-scale deletions have unusual clinical presentations that may be found in the full KSS such as renal tubular acidosis (Eviatar et al., 1990), diabetes/deafness (Dunbar et al., 1993), ataxia/leukodystrophy (Nakai et al., 1994), diabetes–optic atrophy–deafness (Rötig et al., 1993), chronic diarrhoea–villous atrophy (Cormier-Daire et al., 1994), a disease suggesting multiple sclerosis (Bet et al., 1994) and recurrent myoglobinuria (Ohno et al., 1991).

Pearson et al. (1979) described a congenital disorder affecting bone marrow with pancytopenia and altered pancreatic exocrine function. Large-scale deletions were discovered 10 years later by Rötig et al. (1990). This condition may be fatal in infancy but, if the child survives, haematological and pancreatic functions improve to full recovery and the patient develops features of KSS (Blaw & Mize, 1990).

Neurogenic atrophy, ataxia, retinitis pigmentosa (NARP) and maternally inherited Leigh syndrome (MILS)

Holt et al. (1990) first described NARP in adults of a family with maternally inherited symptoms of neurogenic atrophy, ataxia, and retinitis pigmentosa. They found a point mutation at nt 8993 (T→C) in the structural gene for subunit 6 of adenosine triphosphatase synthetase (ATPase). Later, this mutation was found in children with maternally inherited Leigh syndrome (Tautch et al., 1992; Santorelli et al., 1992). Recently, a different mutation was found (T→G) at the same nt 8993 in children with Leigh syndrome (DeVries et al., 1993), and another mutation, corresponding to the same subunit 6 of ATPase, in a mild form of Leigh syndrome at nt 9176 (Thyagarajan et al., 1995).

Cardiomyopathies

A disorder dominated by dilated cardiomyopathy (CMP) and maternally inherited adult-onset myopathy (MIMyCa) was first described by Zeviani et al. (1991) who described a new point mutation at nt 3260 in the tRNA$^{Leu(UUR)}$ gene. Another different mutation in the same gene, at nt 3303, was found in another family with CMP and myopathy; the proband and two siblings had a fatal CMP, and in three maternal relatives the disease was manifested later in life as sudden cardiac death or CMP and myopathy (Silvestri et al., 1994). Two other different mutations in different genes have been reported in association with predominant hypertrophic CMP: (a) a mutation at nt 4269 (A→G) in the tRNA ^{Ile} gene was described in a familial hypertrophic CMP (HCMP) (Tanike et al., 1992); (b) a maternally inherited HCMP in two siblings, one of whom died at 8 months of fatal ventricular arrhythmia (Merante et al., 1994). Hypertrophic CMP was also reported in a relatively large number of patients with MELAS and less frequently in those with MERFF syndrome, although encephalomyopathy was dominating in these conditions.

Leber hereditary optic neuropathy (LHON)

Leber hereditary optic neuropathy (LHON) is characterized mainly by bilateral acute or subacute visual loss in a young adult (18–30 years). Associated features may be cerebellar ataxia, peripheral neuropathy, pre-excitation cardiac syndrome, hyperrreflexia (Di Mauro & Moraes, 1993). Disc oedema and subtle alterations of the retinal vessels are important observations. The first mutation was found at nt11778 (G→A) in the ND4 gene, encoding subunit 4 of complex I (Wallace et al., 1988). LHON is now associated with at least 10 other point mutations in different structural mtDNA genes including ND1, ND2, ND5, cytochrome b of complex III and COX, subunit 1 (see *Neuromuscular Disorders* for an updated review). There is a male predominance in this syndrome and apparently there is a X-linked factor that modulates the expression of mtDNA defect (Bu & Rotter, 1991; Vilkki et al., 1991). Peculiar syndromes associated with LHON mutations are: multiple sclerosis (Harding et al., 1992) or infantile bilateral striatal necrosis with progressive dystonia (Jun et al., 1994).

II. Clinical syndromes with defects in intergenomic communication

Two conditions have been described in which mtDNA defects are the result of a primary molecular defect involving the nDNA.

The first is a dominantly inherited mitochondrial myopathy with PEO, multiple mtDNA deletions and RRF, described by Zeviani et al. (1989). The clinical spectrum of multiple mtDNA deletions has widened since the first description of a myopathy with PEO and tissue specific (muscle) multiple mtDNA deletions (Servidei et al., 1991). Other clinical syndromes with multiple mtDNA deletions include: (a) mitochondrial familial myopathy with probable autosomal recessive (AR) inheritance (Yuzaki *et al.*, 1989); (b) early childhood recurrent ketoacidotic coma or incoordination–drowsiness (Cormier *et al.*, 1991); (c) AR mitochondrial neurogastrointestinal encephalopathy (MNGIE), characterized by a mitochondrial myopathy with RRF, leukoencephalopathy, intestinal pseudo-obstructions and peripheral neuropathy (Uncini *et al.*, 1994); (d) familial recurrent myoglobinuria (Ohno *et al.*, 1991); (f) familial dilated CMP (Suomalainen *et al.*, 1992).

The second condition was reported by Moraes *et al.* (1991) and was defined as a progressive quantitative reduction of mtDNA(depletion). The disease appears to be inherited as an AR trait and intrafamilial tissue expression may be variable within the same kinship. In a review of 10 cases, two phenotypes have been reported (Ricci *et al.*, 1992): (a) a fatal congenital syndrome (7/10) with myopathy (5/7); lactic acidosis (5/7), RRF (5/7), increased creatin kinase (5/7), cardiopathy (2/7), encephalopathy with seizures (2/7), tubular nephropathy (De Toni–Debré–Fanconi) (2/10); isolated liver failure (2/7) (Mazziotta *et al.*, 1992); (b) infantile-onset myopathy (3/10) with increased CK (3/3) and muscle exercise intolerance. A recent study has demonstrated that mtDNA depletion is controlled by the nDNA (Bodnar *et al.*, 1993).

III. Clinical syndromes with probable defects in nDNA

In the past few years most of the progress has been in the area of mDNA genetics where several mtDNA mutations have been associated with specific diseases. In comparison, our understanding of mitochondrial disorders due to nDNA lesions is only preliminary, and molecular defects of nuclear genes have been documented in only few patients; in most cases, defects of the nDNA are only postulated.

Myopathies

Mitochondrial myopathies are generally characterized by muscle weakness or intolerance to exercise. Myopathic syndromes with intolerance to exercise followed by fixed weakness with onset in childhood or in adult life have been associated with defects in complex I and III (Di Mauro & Moraes, 1993). Two forms of myopathy have been associated with complex IV deficiency (Di Mauro *et al.*, 1993): (a) the fatal infantile form (Fig. 1E), that causes respiratory failure and progressive hypotonia, is often associated with a De Toni–Debre–Fanconi syndrome (glycosuria, phosphaturia and aminoaciduria) – a highly inbred family has been described with this form, confirming AR mode of inheritance (Eshel *et al.*, 1991); (b) a benign reversible infantile tissue-specific myopathy that improves spontaneously to normal muscle strength by the age of 2–3 years.

Cardiomyopathies

Mitochondrial disorders with prominent cardiopathy have been reviewed recently (Servidei *et al.*, 1994). Heart involvement in RCD is generally characterized by hypertrophic cardiomyopathy (CMP). In complex I deficiency CMP has been reported, particularly in the multisystemic fatal infantile form; isolated CMP and complex III has been observed in only one infant with peculiar morphological abnormalities classified as 'histiocytoid cardiopathy'. Hypertrophic CMP and complex IV (COX) deficiency has been found to be associated with some cases of fatal infantile myopathy; only one patient has been published with isolated CMP (Kennaway *et al.*, 1990). Recently, hypertrophic CMP in children was studied using endomyocardial biopsies for biochemical detection of RCD, especially in patients with isolated cardiopathy due to possible tissue-specific RCD (Rustin *et al.* 1993, 1994).

Barth syndrome is an X-linked disorder characterized by dilated CMP and myopathy of variable severity (usually fatal in childhood), neutropenia, and 3-methylglutaconic aciduria (Kelley et al., 1991); no definite biochemical marker of this condition has been established and it has been localized to distal Xq28 (Adès et al., 1993).

Three more syndromes with hypertrophic CMP and presumably AR inheritance have been confirmed by several reports of familial cases: (a) cardiopathy and myopathy with combined complex I and IV deficiency (Zheng et al., 1990; Tulinius et al., 1989); (b) 3-methylglutaconic aciduria–mitochondrial myopathy and cardiopathy–multiple respiratory-chain defects, particularly ATP synthase deficiency (complex IV) (Holme et al., 1992; Servidei et al., 1993); (c) Sengers syndrome, characterized by congenital hypotonia, cataracts, easy fatiguability, progressive obstructive CMP with a short PQ interval, and lactic acidosis (Sengers et al., 1984). In one case with Sengers syndrome a combined defect of complex 1 and IV has been found (Servidei et al., 1990).

Encephalomyopathies

The best known and most frequent mitochondrial encephalopathy is Leigh syndrome, a distinctive neuropathological entity defined for its characteristic regional distribution and histopathological features by Leigh in 1951. Lesions are symmetrically distributed in subcortical structures with preferential involvement of the mid-brain, pons, basal ganglia, thalamus and optic nerves, and consist of cystic cavitation, vascular proliferation, neuronal loss, and demyelination. Clinical symptoms include ataxia, strabismus, muscle weakness, respiratory distress and movement disorders (Macaya et al., 1993). In recent years, clinical symptoms, biochemical findings and neuroimaging correlations have allowed the possibility of defining Leigh syndrome before death (Medina et al., 1990). Four major causes are well established by several reports: (a) pyruvate dehydrogenase deficiency transmitted by an AR or X-linked recessive trait depending on the subunit involved (E1α, E1, E2, or E3); (b) AR inheritance with complex IV (COX) deficiency and no RRF (Fig. 1D) (Van Coster et al., 1991); (c) maternally inherited point mutation at 8993 in the ATPase 6 gene of mtDNA (see above); (d) complex I deficiency (Morris et al., 1996).

Other encephalomyopathies have been associated with complex I, complex III and complex IV (Di Mauro & Moraes, 1993). Two main clinical syndomes have been described with complex I deficiency: (a) a fatal infantile multisystem disorder with severe congenital lactic acidosis, hypotonia and weakness, mental retardation and cardiorespiratory failure; (b) mitochondrial encephalomyopathy with onset in childhood or adult life with pleomorphic symptoms including seizures, ophalmoplegia, dementia, ataxia, neurosensory hearing loss, pigmentary retinopathy, neuropathy, movement disorders.

Some rare cases of encephalomyopathy have been associated with complex III deficiency. In addition to Leigh syndrome, COX deficiency has also been found in one case of Alpers syndrome, i.e. progressive poliodystrophy (Prick et al., 1983). A peculiar familial disorder has been associated with coenzyme Q_{10} deficiency in the muscle biopsy of two sisters with slowly progressive weakness, exercise intolerance, recurrent myoglobinuria, and central nervous dysfunction with seizures and ataxia (Ogasahara et al., 1989). This disease is interesting because it may improve after coenzyme Q_{10} supplementation. Two other encephalomyopathies should be briefly described because the pathogenesis is probably related to a defect in mt protein importation: (a) an infantile fatal multisystemic disorder with a deficiency of heat shock protein 60 (Agsteribbe et al., 1993); (b) a pure congenital myopathy with rapid progression at the age of 13 associated with a defect of the iron–sulphur protein of complex III ('Rieskie' protein) and of the 27.2-kD subunit of SDH (Schapira et al., 1990).

References

Adès, L.C., Gedeon, A.K., Wilson, M.J., Latham, M., Partington, M.W., Mulley, J.C., Nelson, J., Lui K. & Sillence D.O. (1993): Barth syndrome: clinical features and confirmation of gene localisation to distal Xq28. *Am. J. Med. Genet.* **45**, 327–334.

Agsteribbe, E., Huckriede, A., Veenhuis, M., Ruiters, M.H., Niezen-Koning, K.E., Skjeldal, O.H., Skullerud, K., Gupta, R.S., Hallberg, R. & van Diggelen, O.P. (1993): A fatal, systemic mitochondrial disease with decreased mitochondrial enzyme activities, abnormal ultrastructure of the mitochondria and deficiency of heat shock protein 60. *Biochem. Biophys. Res. Commun.* **28**, 146–154.

Baumgartner, E.R., Suormala, T.M., Wick, H., Probst, A., Blauenstein, U., Bachmann, C. & Vest, M. (1989): Biotinidase deficiency: a case of subacute necrotizing encephalomyelopathy (Leigh syndrome). Report of a case with lethal outcome. *Pediatr. Res.* **26**, 260–266.

Bennett, M.J., Sherwood, W.G., Gibson, K.M. & Burlina, A.B. (1993): Secondary inhibition of multiple NAD-requiring dehydrogenase in respiratory chain complex I deficiency: possible metabolic markers for the primary defects. *J. Inherit. Metab. Dis.* **16**, 560–562.

Bet, L., Moggio, M., Comi, G.P., Mariani, C., Prelle, A., Checcarelli, N., Bordoni, A., Bresolin, N., Scarpini, E. & Scarlato, G. (1994): Multiple sclerosis and mitochondrial myopathy: an unusual combination of diseases. *J. Neurol.* **241**, 511–516.

Bodnar, A.G., Cooper, J.M., Holt, I.J., Leonard, J.V. & Schapira, A.H.V. (1993): Nuclear complementation restores mtDNA levels in cultured cells from a patient with mtDNA depletion. *Am. J. Hum. Genet.* **53**, 663–669.

Bonnefont, J.P., Specola, N.B., Vassault, A., Lombes, A., Ogier, H., deKlerk, J.B.C., Munnich, A., Coude, M., Paturneau-Jonas, M. & Saudubray, J.M. (1990): The fasting test in paediatrics: application to the diagnosis of pathological hypo-hyperchetotic states. *Eur. J. Pediatr.* **150**, 80–85.

Blaw, M.E. & Mize, C.E. (1990): Juvenile Pearson syndrome. *J. Child. Neurol.* **5**, 187–190.

Bu, X.D. & Rotter, J.I. (1991): X chromosome-linked and mitochondrial gene control of Leber hereditary optic neuropathy: evidence from segregation analysis for dependence on X chromosome inactivation. *Proc. Natl. Acad. Sci. USA* **88**, 8198–8202.

Burlina, A.B., Dionisi-Vici, C., Bennett, M.J., Gibson, K.M., Servidei, S., Bertini, E., Hale, D.E., Schmidt-Sommerfeld, E., Sabetta, G., Zacchello, F. & Rinaldo P. (1994): A new syndrome with ethylmalonic aciduria and normal fatty acid oxidation in fibroblasts. *J. Pediatr.* **124**, 79–86.

Calabresi, P.A., Silvestri, G., Di Mauro, S. & Griggs, R.C. (1994): Ekbom's syndrome: lipomas, ataxia and neuropathy with MERFF. *Muscle Nerve* **17**, 943–945.

Cormier, V., Rötig, A., Tardieu, M., Colonna, M., Saudubray, J.M. & Munnich, A. (1991): Autosomal dominant deletions of the mitochondrial genome in a case of progressive encephalomyopathy. *Am. J. Hum. Genet.* **48**, 643–648.

Cormier-Daire, V., Bonnefont, J.P., Rustin, P., Maurage, C., Ogler, H., Schmitz, J., Ricour, C., Saudubray, J.M., Munnich, A. & Rötig, A. (1994): Mitochondrial DNA rearrangements with onset as chronic diarrhoea with villous atrophy. *J. Pediatr.* **124**, 63–70.

Detre, J.A., Wang, Z., Bogdan, A.R., Gusnard, D.A., Bay, C.A., Bingham, P.M. & Zimmermann, R.A. (1991): Regional variation in brain lactate in Leigh syndrome by localized ^{1}H magnetic resonance spectroscopy. *Ann. Neurol.* **29**, 218–221.

De Vivo, D.C. (1993): The expanding clinical spectum of mitochondrial diseases. *Brain Dev.* **15**, 1–22.

De Vries, D.D., van Engelen, B.G.M., Gabrieels, F.J.M., Ruitenbeek, W. & van Oost, B.A. (1993): A second missense mutation in mitochondrial ATPase 6 gene in Leigh syndrome. *Ann. Neurol.* **34**, 410–412.

Di Mauro, S. (1993): Mitochondrial encephalomyopathies. In: *The molecular and genetic basis of neurological disease*, eds. R.H. Rosemberg, S.B. Prusiner, S. Di Mauro et al., pp 665–694. Boston: Butterworth-Heinemann.

Di Mauro, S. & Moraes, C. (1993): Mitochondrial encephalomyopathies. *Arch. Neurol.* **50**, 1197–1208.

Di Mauro, S., Hirano, M., Bonilla, E., Moraes, C.T. & Schon, E.A. (1993): Cytochrome oxidase deficiency: progress and problems. In: *The molecular and genetic basis of neurological disease*, eds. R.H. Rosemberg, S.B Prusiner, S. Di Mauro et al., pp. 91–115. Boston: Butterworth-Heinemann.

Dunbar, D.R., Moonie, P.A., Swingler, R.J., Davidson, D., Roberts, R. & Holt, I.J. (1993): Maternally transmitted partial direct tandem duplication of mitochondrial DNA associated with diabetes mellitus. *Hum. Mol. Genet.* **2**, 1619–1624.

Engel, W.K. & Cunningham, G.G. (1963): Rapid examination of muscle tissue: an improved trichrome stain method for frozen biopsy sections. *Neurology* **13**, 919–926.

Eshel, G., Lahat, E., Fried, K., Barr, J., Barosh, V., Gutman, A., Di Mauro, S. & Aladjem, M. (1991): Autosomal recessive lethal infantile cytochrome C oxidase deficiency. *A.J.D.C.* **145**, 661–664.

Eviatar, L., Shanske, S., Gauthier, B., Abrams, C., Maytal, J., Slavin, M., Valderrama, E. & Di Mauro, S. (1990): Kearns–Sayre syndrome presenting as renal tubular acidosis. *Neurology* **40**, 1761–1763.

Fukuhara, N., Tokiguchi, S., Shirakawa, H. & Tsubaki, T. (1980): Myoclonus epilepsy associated with ragged-red fibers (mitochondrial abnormalities). Disease entity or a syndrome? Light and electronmicroscopic studies of two cases and review of the literature. *J. Neurol. Sci.* **47**, 117–133.

Gibson, K.M., Bennett, M.J., Mize, C.E., Jakobs, C., Rötig, A., Munnich, A., Lichter Konecki, U. & Trefz, F.K. (1992): 3-methyglutaconic aciduria associated with Pearson syndrome and respiratory chain defects. *J. Pediatr.* **121**, 940–942.

Goto, Y-I., Nonaka, I. & Horai, S. (1990): A mutation in the tRNA$^{Leu(UUR)}$ gene associated with the MELAS sub-group of mitochondrial encephalomyopathies. *Nature* **348**, 651–653.

Hasegawa, H., Matsuoka, T., Goto, Y-I. & Nonaka, I. (1991): Strongly succinate dehydrogenase-reactive blood vessels in muscles from patients with mitochondrial myopathy, encephalopathy, lactic acidosis and stroke-like episodes. *Ann. Neurol.* **29**, 610–605.

Harding, A.E., Sweeney, M.G., Miller, D.H., Mumford, C.J., Kellar-Wod, H., Menard, D., McDonald, W.I. & Compston, A.S. (1992): Occurence of a multiple sclerosis-like illness in women who have a Leber's hereditary optic neuropathy mitochondrial DNA mutation. *Brain* **115**, 979–989.

Hirano, M., Ricci, E., Koenigsberger, M.R., Defendini, R., Pavlakis, S.G., De Vivo, D.C., Di Mauro, S. & Rowland, L.P. (1992): MELAS: original case and clinical criteria for diagnosis. *Neuromusc. Disord.* **2**, 125–135.

Hirano, M. & Pavlakis, S.G. (1994): Mitochondrial myopathy, encephalopathy, lactic acidosis, and stroke-like episodes (MELAS): current concepts. *J. Child. Neurol.* **9**, 4–13.

Holme, E., Greter, J. & Jacobson, C.E. (1992): Mitochondrial ATP-synthase deficiency in a child with 3-methylglutaconic aciduria. *Pediatr. Res.* **32**, 731–735.

Holt, I.J., Harding, A.E. & Morgan-Hughes, J.A. (1988): Deletions of muscle mitochondrial DNA in patients with mitochondrial myopathies. *Nature* **331**, 717–719.

Jakobs, C., Danse, P. & Veermann, A.J.P. (1991): Organic aciduria in Pearson syndrome. *Eur. J. Pediatr.* **150**, 684.

Johns, D.R., Plotkin, G.M., Logigian, E.L. & Sudarsky, L.R. (1994): Dystonia as manifestation of the 3243 mtDNA mutation. *Ann. Neurol.* **36**, 315 (abstract).

Jun, A.S., Brown, M.D. & Wallace, D.C. (1994): A mitochondrial DNA mutation at nucleotide pair 14459 of the NADH dehydrogenase subunit 6 gene associated with maternally inherited Leber hereditary optic neuropathy and dystonia. *Proc. Natl. Acad. Sci. USA* **91**, 6206–6210.

Kearns, T.P. & Sayre, G.P. (1958): Retinitis pigmentosa, external opthalmoplegia, and complete heart block. *Ophthalmology* **60**, 280–289.

Kelley, R.I., Cheatham, J.P. & Clark, B.J. (1991): X-linked dilated cardiomyopathy with neutropenia, growth retardation, and 3-methylglutaconic aciduria. *J. Pediatr.* **119**, 738–747.

Kennaway, N.G., Carrero-Valenzuela, R.D., Ewart, G., Balan, V.K., Lightowlers, R., Zhang, Y.Z., Powell, B.R., Capaldi, R.A. & Buist, N.R. (1990): Isoforms of mammalian cytochrome c oxidase deficiency with human cytochrome c oxidase deficiency. *Pediatr. Res.* **28**, 529–535.

Leigh, D. (1951): Subacute necrotizing encephalomyelopathy in an infant. *J. Neurol. Neurosurg. Psychiatry* **14**, 216–221.

Lodi, R., Montagna, P., Iotti, S., Zanoil, P., Barboni, P., Puddu, P. & Barbirolli, B. (1994): Brain and muscle energy metabolism studied in vivo by ^{31}P-magnetic resonance spectroscopy in NARP syndrome. *J. Neurol. Neurosurg. Psychiatry* **57**, 1492–1496.

Macaya, A., Munell, F., Burke, R.E. & De Vivo, D.C. (1993): Disorders of movement in Leigh syndrome. *Neuropediatrics* **24**, 60–67.

Mathews, P.M., Andermann, F., Silver, K., Karpati, G. & Arnold, D.L. (1994): Proton MR spectroscopic characterization of differences in regional brain metabolic abnormalities in mitochondrial encephalomyopathies. *Neurology* **43**, 2482–2490.

Mazziotta, M.R., Ricci, E., Bertini, E., Dionisi-Vici, C., Servidei, S., Burlina, A.B., Sabetta, G., Bartuli, A., Manfredi, G. & Silvestri, G. (1992): Fatal infantile liver failure associated with mitochondrial DNA depletion. *J. Pediatr.* **121**, 896–901.

Medina, L., Chi, T.L, De Vivo, D.C. & Hilal, S.K. (1990): MR manifestations of biochemically characterized subacute necrotizing encephalomyelopathy (Leigh syndrome): genetic evidence for a nuclear DNA-encoded mutation. *Neurology* **39**, 697–702.

Merante, F., Tein, I., Benson, L. & Robinson, B.H. (1994): Maternally inherited hypertrophic cardiomyopathy due to a novel T→C transition at nucleotide 9997 in the mitochondrial tRNA^{glycine} gene. *Am. J. Hum. Genet.* **55**, 437–446.

Moraes, C.T., Shanske, S., Trischeler, H.J., Aprille, J.R., Andreetta, F., Bonilla, E., Schon, E.A. & Di Mauro, S. (1991): mtDNA depletion with variable tissue expression: a novel genetic abnormality in mitochondrial diseases. *Am. J. Hum. Genet.* **48**, 492–501.

Moraes, C.T., Ciacci, F., Silvestri, G., Shanske, S., Sciacco, M., Hirano, M., Schon, E.A., Bonilla, E. & Di Mauro, S. (1993): Atypical clinical presentations associated with the MELAS mutation at position 3243 of human mitochondrial DNA. *Neuromusc. Disord.* **3**, 43–50.

Morris, A.A.M., Leonard, J.V., Brown, G.K., Bidouki, S.K., Bindoff, L.A., Woodward, C.E., Harding, A.E., Farrell, M.A., Bell, J.E., Minekhun, M. & Turnbull, D.M. (1996): Deficiency of respiratory chain complex 1 is a common cause of Leigh disease. *Ann. Neurol.* **40**, 25–30.

Nakai, A., Goto, Y., Fujisawa, K., Shigematsu, Y., Kikawa, Y., Konishi, Y., Nonaka, I. & Sudo, M. (1994): Diffuse leukodystrophy with large-scale mitochondrial DNA deletion. *Lancet* **343**, 1397–1398.

Nashef, L. & Lane, R.J. (1989): Screening for mitochondrial cytopathies: the sub-anaerobic threshold exercise test (SATET). *J. Neurol. Neurosurg. Psychiatry* **52**, 1090–1094.

Ogasahara, S., Engel, A.G., Frens, D. & Mack, D. (1989): Muscle coezyme Q deficiency in a familial mitochondrial encephalomyopathy. *Proc. Natl. Acad. Sci. USA* **86**, 2379–2384.

Ohno, K., Tanaka, M., Sahashi K., Ibi, Sato, W., Yamamoto, T. & Takahashi (1991): Mitochondrial DNA deletions in inherited recurrent myoglobinuria. *Ann. Neurol.* **29**, 364–369.

Pavlakis, S.G., Rowland, L.P., De Vivo, D.C., Bonilla, E. & Di Mauro, S. (1988): Mitochondrial myopathies and encephalomyopathies. In: *Advances in contemporary neurology,* ed. F. Plum, pp. 95–133. New York: F.A. Davis.

Pearson, H.A, Lobel, J.S., Kocoshis, S.A, Naiman, J.L., Windmiller, J., Lammi, A.T. & Hoffman, R. (1979): A new syndrome of refractory sideroblastic anemia with vacuolization of marrow precursors and exocrine pancreatic dysfunction. *J. Pediatr.* **95**, 976–984.

Perry, T.L., Hansen, S., Booth, F.A., Penn, A.M.W., Jones, K. & Dilling, L.A. (1989): An unusual aminoacidopathy associated with mitochondrial encephalomyopathy. *J. Inherit. Metab. Dis.* **12**, 23–32.

Poulton, J., Deadman, M.E. & Gardiner, R.M. (1989): Duplication of mitochondrial DNA in mitochondrial myopathies. *Lancet* **i**, 236–240.

Prick, M.J.J., Gabreels, F.J.M., Trijbels, J.M.F., Janssen, A.J., le Coultre, R., van Dam, K., Jaspar, H.H., Ebels, E.J. & Op de Coul, A.A. (1983): Progressive poliodystrophy (Alpers disease) with defect in cytochrome aa3 in muscle: a report of two unrelated patients. *Clin. Neurol. Neurosurg.* **85**, 57–70.

Ricci, E., Moraes, C., Servidei, S., Tonali, P., Bonilla, E. & Di Mauro, S. (1992): Disorders associated with depletion of mitochondrial DNA. *Brain Pathol.* **2**, 141–147.

Robinson, B.H., Glerum, D.M., Chow, W., Petrova-Benedict, R., Lightowlers, R. & Capaldi, R. (1990): The use of skin fibroblast cultures in the detection of respiratory chain defects in patients with lacticidemia. *Pediatr. Res.* **28**, 549–555.

Robinson, B.H., Petrova-Benedict, R., Buncic, J.R. & Wallace, D.C. (1992): Nonviability of cells with oxidative defects in galactose medium: a screening test for affected patient fibroblasts. *Biochem. Med. Metab. Biol.* **48**, 122–126.

Rötig, A., Colonna, M., Bonnefont, J.P., Ledeist, F., Romero, N., Schmitz, J., Rustin, P., Fischer, A., Saudubray, J.M. & Munnich, A. (1990): Pearson's marrow-pancreas syndrome: a multisystem mitochondrial disorder in infancy. *J. Clin. Invest.* **86**, 1601–1608.

Rötig, A., Cormier, V., Chatelain, P., Francois, R., Saudubray, J.M., Rustin, P. & Munnich, A. (1993): Deletion of mitochondrial DNA in a case of early-onset diabetes mellitus, optic atrophy, and deafness (Wolfram syndrome, MIM 222300). *J. Clin. Invest.* **91**, 1095–1098.

Rowland, L.P., Blake, D.M., Hirano, M., Di Mauro, S., Schon, E.A., Hays, A.P. & De Vivo, D.C. (1991): Clinical syndromes associated with ragged-red fibers. *Rev. Neurol.* **290**, 457.

Rustin, P., Chretien, D., Bourgeron, T., Le Bidois, J., Sidi, D., Rötig, A. & Munnich, A. (1993): Investigation of respiratory chain activity in human heart. *Biochem. Med. Metab. Biol.* **50**, 120–126.

Rustin, P., Lebidois, J., Cretien, D., Burgeron, T., Piechaud, J.F., Rötig, A., Munnich, A. & Sidi, D. (1994): Endomyocardial biopsies for early detection of mitochondrial disorders in hypertrophic cardiomyopathies. *J. Pediatr.* **124**, 224–228.

Santorelli, F., Shanske, S., Macaya, A., De Vivo, D.C. & Di Mauro, S. (1992): The mutation at nt 8993 of mitochondrial DNA is a common cause of Leigh's syndrome. *Ann. Neurol.* **32,** 467–468.

Schapira, A.H.V., Cooper, J.M., Morgan-Hughes, J.A., Landon, D.N. & Clark, J.B. (1990): Mitochondrial myopathy with a defect of mitochondrial-protein transport. *N. Engl. J. Med.* **323,** 37-42.

Senghers, R.C.A., Trijbels, J.M.F., Bakkeren, A.J.M., Ruitenbeck, W., Fischer, J.C., Janssen, A.J.M., Stadhouders, A.M. & Lavak, H.J. (1984): Deficiency of cytochromes b and a3, in muscle from a floppy infant with cytochrome oxidase deficiency. *Eur. J. Pediatr.* **141,** 178–180.

Servidei, S., Dionisi-Vici, C., Bertini, E., Manfredi, G., Silvestri, G., Sabetta, G. & Tonali, P. (1990): Sengers syndrome with deficiency of respiratory complexes I and IV. *Ital. J. Neurol. Sci.* **11,** 194 (abstract).

Servidei, S., Zeviani, M., Manfredi, G., Ricci, E., Silvestri, G., Bertini, E., Gellera, C., Di Mauro, S., Di Donato, S. & Tonali, P. (1991): Dominantly inherited mitochondrial myopathy with multiple deletions of mitochondrial DNA: clinical, morphological, and biochemical studies. *Neurology* **41,** 1053–1059.

Servidei, S., Bertini, E., Manfredi, G., Dionisi-Vici, C., Silvestri, G., Ricci, E., Burlina, A.B. & Tonali, P. (1993): Familial infantile myopathy and cardiomyopathy with deficiency of cytochrome c oxidase (COX) and mitochondrial ATP-synthase (ATP-S). *Ann. Neurol.* **34,** 463–464 (abstract).

Servidei, S., Bertini, E. & Di Mauro, S. (1994): Hereditary metabolic cardiomyopathies. *Adv. Pediatr.* **41,** 1–32.

Silvestri, G., Moraes, C.T., Shanske, S., Oh, S.J. & Di Mauro, S. (1992): A new point mutation in the other tRNA^{Lys} gene associated with myoclonic epilepsy and ragged-red fibers (MERFF). *Am. J. Hum. Genet.* **51,** 1213–1217.

Silvestri, G., Cianfaloni, E., Santarelli, F.M., Shanske, S., Servidei, S., Graf, W.D., Sumi, M. & Di Mauro, S. (1993): Clinical features associated with the A→G transition at the nucleotide 8344 of mtDNA ("MERFF mutation"). *Neurology* **43,** 1200–1206.

Silvestri, G., Santorelli, F.M., Shanske, S.B., Whitley, C.B., Schimmenti, L.A., Smith, S.A. & Di Mauro, S. (1994): A new mitochondrial DNA mutation in the tRNA$^{Leu(UUR)}$ gene associated with cardiomyopathy and ragged red fibers. *Hum. Mut.* **3,** 37–43.

Shoffner, J.M., Lott, M.T., Lezza, A.M.S., Seibel, P., Ballinger, S.W. & Wallace, D.C. (1990): Myoclonic epilepsy and ragged-red fibers (MERFF) is associated with a mitochondrial DNA tRNA^{Lys} gene mutation. *Cell* **348,** 651–653.

Suomalainen, A., Pateau, A., Leinonen, H., Majander, A., Peltonen, L. & Somer, H. (1992): Inherited idiopathic dilated cardiomyopathy with multiple deletions of mitochondrial DNA. *Lancet* **340,** 1319–1320.

Tanike, M., Fukushima, H., Yanagihara, I. *et al.* (1992): Mitochondrial tRNA^{Ile} mutation in fatal cardiomyopathy. *Biochem. Biophys. Res. Commun.* **186,** 47–53.

Tautch, Y., Christodoulou, J., Feigenbaum, A., Clarke, J.T., Wherret, J., Smith, C., Rudd, N., Petova-Benedict, R. & Robinson, B.H. (1992): Heteroplasmic mtDNA mutation (T→G) at 8,993 can cause Leigh disease when the percentage of abnormal mtDNA is high. *Am. J. Hum. Genet.* **50,** 852–858.

Thyagarajan, D., Shonske, S., Vasquez-Munije, M., De Vivo, D. and Di Mauro, S. (1995): A novel mitochondrial ATPase 6 point mutation in familial bilateral striatal necrosis. *Ann. Neurol.* **38,** 468–472.

Trijbels, J.M.F., Sengers, R.C.A., Ruitenbek, W., Fischer, J.C., Bakkeren, J.A.J. & Jansenn, A.J.M. (1988): Disorders of the mitochondrial respiratory chain: clinical manifestations and diagnostic approach. *Eur. J. Pediatr.* **148,** 92–97.

Tulinius, M.H., Eriksson, B.O., Hjalmarsson, O., Holme, E. & Oldorfs, A. (1989): Mitochondrial myopathy and cardiomyopathy in siblings. *Pediatr. Neurol.* **5,** 182–188.

Tzika, A.A., Ball, W.S., Vigneron, D.B., Dunn, R.S. & Kirks, D.R. (1994): Clinical proton MR spectroscopy of neurodegenerative diseases in childhood. *AJNR* **14,** 1267–1281.

Uncini, A., Servidei, S., Silvestri, G., Manfredi, G., Sabatelli, M., Di Muzio, A., Ricci, E., Mirabella, M., Di Mauro, S., & Tonali, P. (1994): Ophthalmoplegia, demyelinating neuropathy, leukoencephalopathy, myopathy, and gastrointestinal dysfunction with multiple deletions of mitochondrial DNA: a mitochondrial multisystem disorder in search of a name. *Muscle Nerve* **17,** 667–674.

Van Coster R., Lombes, A., De Vivo, D.C., Chi, T.L., Dodson, W.E., Rothman, S., Orrechio, E.J., Grover, W., Berry, G.T., Schwartz, J.F., Habib, A. & Di Mauro, S. (1991): Cytochrome c oxidase-associated Leigh syndrome: phenotypic features and pathogenetic speculations. *J. Neurol. Sci.* **104,** 97–111.

Van den Ouweland, J.M.W., Lemkes, H.H.P.J., Tremboth, R.C., Ross, R., Velho, G., Cohen, D., Froguel, P. & Maassen, A. (1994): Maternally inherited diabetes and deafness is a distinct subtype of diabetes and associates with a single point mutation in the mitochondrial tRNA$^{Leu(UUR)}$ gene. *Diabetes* **43,** 746–751.

Vassault, A., Bonnefont, J.P., Specola, N. & Saudubray, J.M. (1991): Lactate, pyruvate, and ketone bodies. In: *Techniques in diagnostic human biochemical genetics: a laboratory manual,* ed. F.A. Hommes, pp. 285–308. New York: Wiley-Liss.

Vilkki, J., Ott, J., Savontaus, M.L., Aula, P. & Nikoskelainen, E.K. (1991): Optic atrophy in Leber hereditary optic neuroretinopathy is probably determined by an X-chromosome gene closely linked to DXS7. *Am. J. Hum.Genet.* **48,** 486–491.

Wallace, D.C., Singh, G., Lott, M.T., Hodge, J.A., Shurr, T.G., Lezza, A.M. & Elsas, L.J. (1988): Mitochondrial DNA mutation associated with Leber's hereditary optic neuropathy. *Science* **242,** 1427–1430.

Wallace, D.C. & Lott, M.Y. (1993): Maternally inherited diseases. In: *Mitochondrial DNA human pathology,* eds. S. Di Mauro & D.C. Wallace, pp. 63–83. New York: Raven Press.

Wanders, R.J., Ruiter, J.P. & Wijiburg, F.A. (1993): Studies on mitochondrial oxidative phosphorylation in permeabilized human skin fibroblasts: application to mitochondrial encephalomyopathies. *Biochim. Biophys. Acta* **1181,** 219–222.

Yuzaki, M., Ohkoshi, N., Kanazawa, I., Kagawa, Y. & Ohta, S. (1989): Multiple deletions in mitochondrial DNA at direct repeats of non-D-loop regions in cases of familial mitochondrial myopathy. *Biochem. Biophys. Res. Commun.* **164,** 1352–1357.

Zheng, X., Shofner, J.M., Lott, M.T., Voljavec, A.S., Krawiecki, N.S., Winn, K. & Wallace, D.C. (1990): Evidence in a lethal infantile mitochondrial disease for a nuclear mutation affecting respiratory complexes I and IV. *Neurology* **39,** 1203–1209.

Zeviani, M., Servidei, S., Gellera, C., Bertini, E., Di Mauro, S. & Di Donato, S. (1989): An autosomal dominant disorder with multiple deletions of mitochondrial DNA starting at the D-loop region. *Nature* **339,** 309–311.

Zeviani, M., Gellera, C., Antozzi, C., Rimoldi, M., Morandi, L., Villani, F., Tiranti, V. & Di Donato, S. (1991): Maternally inherited myopathy and cardiomyopathy: association with mutation in mitochondrial DNA tRNA$^{Leu(UUR)}$. *Lancet* **338,** 143–147.

Zeviani, M., Muntoni, F., Savarese, N., Serra, G., Tiranti, V., Carrara, F., Mariotti, C. & Di Donato, S. (1993): A MERFF/MELAS overlap syndrome with a new point mutation in the mitochondrial other tRNA ^{Lys} gene. *Eur. J. Hum. Genet.* **1,** 80–87.

Chapter 3

Congenital muscular dystrophies

Michel Fardeau,[1] Fernando M.S. Tomé,[1] Anne Helbling-Leclerc,[1] Teresinha Evangelista,[1] Emilia Manole,[1] Alberto Ottolini,[1] Martine Chevallay,[1] Sabine Fauré[2] and Dominique Hillaire[2]

[1]*INSERM U.153, Institut de Myologie, Hôpital de la Salpêtrière, 47 boulevard de l'Hôpital, 75651 Paris;* [2]*Généthon, 1 rue de l'Internationale, 91002 Evry, France*

Summary

Congenital muscular dystrophies (CMD) comprise a highly complex, heterogeneous group of disorders. The description by Fukuyama of a peculiar form frequent in Japan (FCMD) emphasized the importance of CNS involvement in these disorders. Other forms are associated with severe mental and sensory involvement (muscle–eye–brain disease) described in Finland or with the Walker–Warburg syndrome. Brain imaging techniques allowed recognition of the frequency of infraclinical brain abnormalities in occidental, 'classical' CMD.

An important breakthrough in the pathogenesis of CMD came with the discovery of a selective deficiency in a specific laminin isovariant, merosin or laminin 2, made of three chains (M or α 2, B1 or β1 and B2 or γ1). Seventeen out of 36 patients were found to be merosin deficient. Comparison of the clinical data between the two groups, merosin deficient (CMD mer–) and merosin non-deficient (CMD mer+), led to the conclusion that CMD mer– comprises a more homogeneous group of patients than CMD mer+. Similar findings were reported by others.

A genetic linkage with a 6q2 locus, corresponding to M-chain gene localization, was found thanks to a panel of informative families with CMD, of French and Turkish origin. CMD mer+ did not map either onto this locus, or onto the FCMD 9q31–33 locus. Thus, CMD mer– can be considered as a new entity within the group of CMD.

The term congenital muscular dystrophy (CMD) was originally proposed (Howard, 1908) to designate muscular disorders of very early clinical onset, marked weakness and atrophy, multiple contractures and joint deformities, and delayed motor development contrasting with normal mental functions. However, nosological classification of these disorders remained uncertain for several decades, and a number of cases were reported under various titles, such as myatonia congenita, infantile myopathies, congenital myopathies, etc. (see Nonaka & Chou, 1979; Banker, 1994). Histopathological studies of muscle biopsies did not contribute much, as they showed non-specific changes of the muscle fibres, compatible with any dystrophic process (Afifi *et al.*, 1969; Zellweger *et al.*, 1967a, b). The diagnosis of CMD was often accepted after exclusion of the different types of structural congenital myopathies. An autosomal recessive inheritance was generally postulated. It was clear, from the different series observed in Western countries, that a marked clinical heterogeneity existed in this group, and some cases were considered distinct enough to be described apart, such as the atonic-sclerotic syndrome (Ullrich, 1930), or some cases were identified as rigid spine syndromes (Dubowitz, 1973).

In 1960, a peculiar form of CMD (FCMD) was reported in Japan by Fukuyama, which was characterized by the association of muscle dystrophy with severe CNS disturbances. The disease was generally very severe, the highest motor level reached by the children being generally crawling on the buttocks or the knees, and in addition, they had a very low IQ often associated with epilepsy. CT scans showed decreases in the density of the white matter, ventricular dilatation and cortical atrophy; neuropathological examination revealed consistently marked changes, with pachygyria or micropolygyria of the cerebral and cerebellar cortex (Fukuyama et al., 1981; Osawa et al., 1991). Several hundred of such children were detected in Japan, and only very few outside. An autosomal recessive inheritance was rapidly considered to be highly probable (Osawa, 1978).

A few years later, in Finland, Santavuori et al. (1977) reported a series of cases in which the muscle disorder was associated with severe brain and eye changes – hence the name muscle–eye–brain (MEB) disease. In parallel, muscle dystrophic lesions were reported in children presenting with the Walker–Warburg syndrome (WWS) (Dobyns et al. 1989), a lethal autosomal recessive disease with cobblestone lissencephaly and ocular (mainly retinal) malformations (Pavone et al., 1986; Lichtig et al., 1993). The relationship between MEB disease and WWS is still disputed. But all these descriptions pointed out the frequent association of CMD with brain and sensory abnormalities.

In Western countries, CMD usually presents as pure muscular disorder with a normal intellectual development (Donner et al., 1975; Serratrice et al., 1980). However, when non-invasive techniques of brain imaging were available, white matter changes were also detected in a significant proportion of CMD (Bernier et al., 1979; Egger et al., 1983; Echenne et al., 1986; Trevisan et al., 1991). Thus, CMD appeared as a more complex entity than it was thought from the early reports.

Another important feature which was striking for any pathologist looking at CMD muscle biopsies was the marked increase of endomysial connective tissue, contrasting with the relative discreteness of muscle fibre changes, except in the early stages of the disease where necrotic and regenerative changes were observed. This led researchers to consider that the '*primum movens*' of the dystrophies could be located in the extracellular matrix (Fidzianska et al., 1982). Early studies failed to detect any qualitative abnormalities in collagen components (Duance et al., 1980; Hantaï et al., 1985).

The discovery, by Campbell and his group (Campbell & Kahl, 1989; Ervasti & Campbell, 1991; Ibraghimov-Beskrovnaya et al., 1992), of a large oligomeric complex of sarcolemmal proteins associated with dystrophin, providing a link between intracellular cytoskeleton and extracellular proteins such as laminin, led to reinvestigation of this hypothesis, checking whether one of the laminin isoforms could be involved in these dystrophies. Laminin is an heterotrimer, made up of three chains arranged in various combinations, and several variants were described (Engvall, 1993). The laminin variant present in nerve and muscle basement membrane was named merosin or laminin 2, with an M (or $\alpha 2$) chain associated with B_1 (or $\beta 1$) and B_2 (or $\gamma 1$) chains (Leivo & Engvall, 1988; Ehrig et al., 1990; Burgeson et al., 1994). Antibodies raised against these different chains allowed immunocytochemical studies in CMD biopsies to be undertaken.

In FCMD, sarcolemmal labelling with anti-dystrophin antibodies, as well as with anti-laminin antibodies, showed some diminution and irregularities (Arikawa et al., 1991; Hayashi et al., 1993). Systematic analysis of a series of 'classical' CMD led to the surprising discovery that merosin was completely deficient in some cases, whereas the A chain was overexpressed (Fig. 1); the B_1 and B_2 chains had a normal level of expression (Tomé et al., 1994). This was confirmed by immunoblotting techniques.

About half of the CMD biopsies showed merosin deficiency. A series of 15 cases was initially reported (Fardeau & Tomé, 1994) and this finding was soon confirmed by other groups (Philpot et al., 1995; Topaloglu et al., 1994). Several other cases were detected, and our personal series includes 17 merosin-deficient cases out of 36 cases diagnosed as CMD.

Chapter 3   Congenital muscular dystrophies

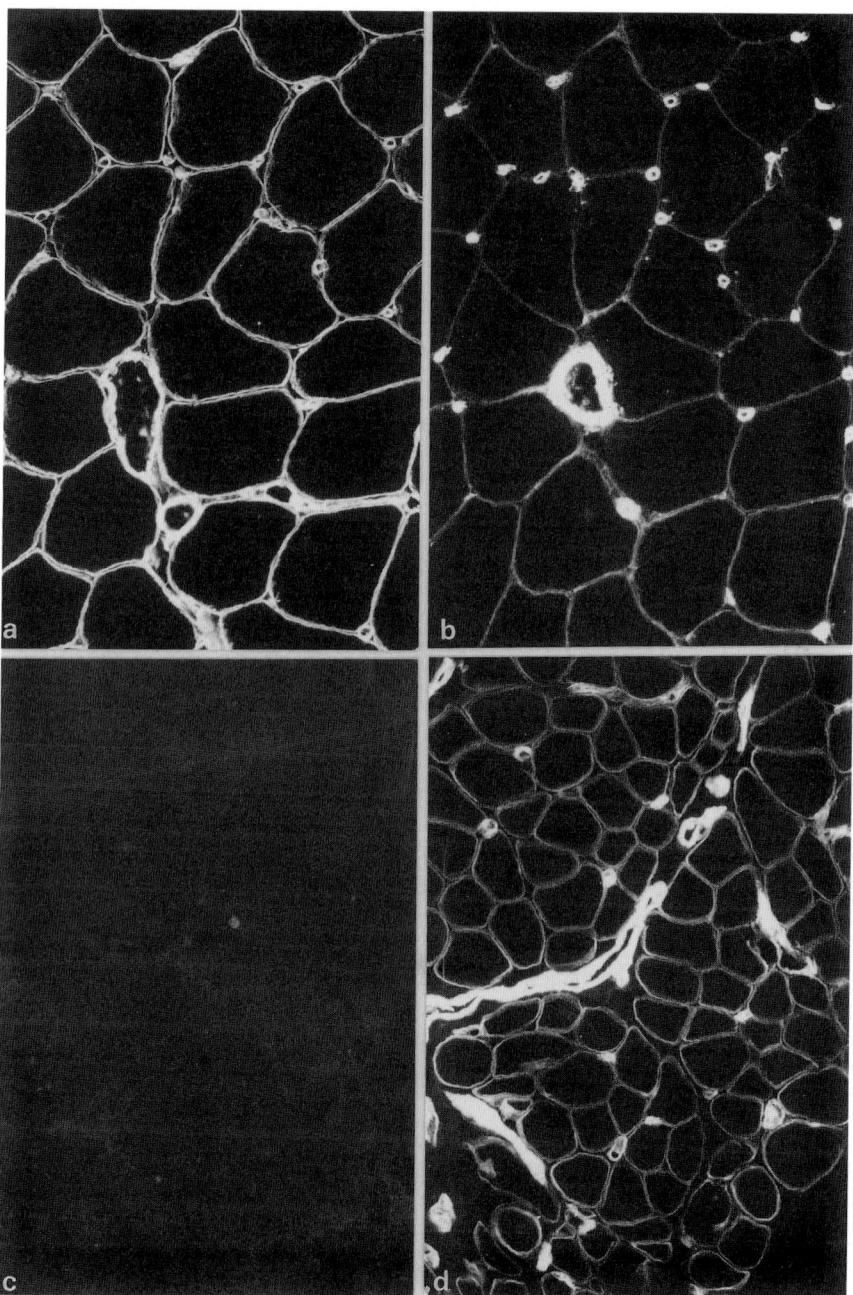

Fig. 1. Immunocytochemical analysis of merosin (a and c), and laminin A chain (b and d) in serial sections of muscle biopsies from a normal control (a and b) and 8-month-old child with congenital muscular dystrophy (c and d). The normal strong expression of merosin (a) and the very weak expression of the laminin A chain (b) around muscle fibres; laminin A chain is normally strongly expressed in the basal lamina of blood vessels. In a child with congenital muscular dystrophy there is no merosin (c) and overexpression of the laminin A chain (d) around muscle fibres. Magnification × 235.

Interestingly, the comparison of the clinical data of the merosin-deficient cases with the non-deficient led us to consider that the merosin-deficient group was more homogeneous that the non-deficient group. Merosin-deficient patients (Table 1) had generally a more severe presentation, with a marked and constant neonatal hypotonia, and multiple and early contractures: only 3/17 were able to walk with support; a severe respiratory insufficiency needing ventilatory assistance was present in four patients. Most (7/8) of the children explored by CT scan or MRI showed white matter changes. It is noticeable that in two patients, brain images were considered normal in their early months and definitely abnormal a few years later. Mental development was generally considered normal, but epileptic seizures were present in two patients. The severity of the disease is illustrated by the fact that 5/17 died before 10 years of age.

Table 1. 'Merosin-deficient' CMD

17 cases (10 M, 7 F)		
Hypotonia	Most often marked or severe in the neonatal period	(12/17)
Contractures	Multiple and severe	(14/17)
Motor development	Markedly delayed; did not walk	(13/17) (6/14)*
Respiratory insufficiency	Frequent, sometimes severe	(4/13)
Mental development	Usually normal	(13/15)
Brain abnormalities (MRI scan)	Frequent	(7/8)
Serum CK	Markedly raised in the early stages	(13/14)
Evolution	Severe	5 died before 10 years

* 3 died before normal walking age.

By contrast, the merosin non-deficient cases (Table 2) were generally of less severity. Neonatal hypotonia was rarely marked. Contractures were constant, but rarely severe and often delayed. Motor development was rarely severely delayed; 14 out of 19 children were able to walk. It should be noticed, however, that a progression of the weakness was observed in some children after a few years. Respiratory insufficiency was present only in four patients. Mental development was considered normal in most cases, but retarded in three children. In four patients explored by MRI, no brain abnormalities were found. Furthermore, this group of merosin non-deficient CMD patients exhibited a marked clinical heterogeneity. Two children were considered as having possible Ullrich syndrome, with marked distal hyperextensibility; one child presented with a curious and marked scapular and pelvic muscular hypertrophy before the wasting process had occurred.

Table 2. 'Merosin non-deficient' CMD

19 cases (8 M, 11 F)		
Hypotonia	Rarely severe	(6/19)
Contractures	Rarely severe	(2/19)
Motor development	Usually delayed; did not walk	(5/19)
Respiratory insufficiency	Infrequent, rarely severe	(4/15)
Mental development	Usually normal	(16/19)
Brain abnormalities	Rare (?)	(0/4)
Serum CK	Markedly raised in the early stage	(10/16)
Evolution	Rarely severe	1 died (neonatal period)

Similar data, with the same characteristics, were noticed in the British and Turkish series (Topaloglu et al., 1994; Philpot et al., 1995). Taken together, these results highly suggest that the merosin-deficient CMD (CMD mer–) forms a homogeneous entity. This was corroborated by the genetic studies. As the preceding data suggested that laminin Mα2 chain could be a candidate for causing the disease, a genetic study was undertaken on a panel of four CMD mer– consanguinous families and compared to a panel of three merosin non-deficient (CMD mer+) families. Homozygosity mapping and linkage analysis were performed; two loci were checked, on chromosome 6q2, where the Mα2 chain gene was localized (Vuolteenaho et al., 1994), and on chromosome 9q31–33, where the FCMD gene was mapped, after the discovery of a child presenting both FCMD and xeroderma pigmentosum – previously localized in this locus (Toda et al., 1993). The results were positive for the 6q2 locus, and these studies allowed the localization of the CMD mer– gene on a 16 cM region of the locus, with a lod score of 5.56 for $\Theta = 0$ (Hillaire et al., 1994). Exclusion figures were found for the merosin non-deficient group. This study also allowed the exclusion of any linkage of this group with the 9q31–33 locus. Mutations have subsequently been discovered in the laminin a2-chain (or M chain) gene (Helbling-Leclerc et al., 1995).

CMDs are now becoming clarified, and no one could imagine two years ago how fast things would run in this complex field. Moreover, the discovery of a merosin deficiency in CMD may lead to several important new developments.

The first development concerns the merosin non-deficient CMDs. Molecular genetic studies should be undertaken in the different subsets of these dystrophies. Furthermore, it should be emphasized that a few cases are characterized by an incomplete and variable deficiency in merosin, sometimes with evidence of leukoencephalopathy (Trevisan et al., 1995), suggesting that merosin deficiency might be partial, or secondary to another membrane-protein defect. CMD partial merosin deficiencies have been localized on the same LAMA2 gene, and causal mutations identified (Helbling-Leclerc, Topaloglu et al., 1995; Nissinen et al., 1996).

The second deals with the mechanism of the disease. It is indeed intriguing that the necrotic–regenerative pattern of the disease is rapidly burn out. This might be related to the low number and inactive state of the satellite cells in this dystrophy (Fardeau et al., 1978), as compared, for instance, with Duchenne's dystrophy. An activating role of merosin upon myogenic cells should be explored.

The third is the possibility of an original method of prenatal diagnosis. Merosin is present in the placenta, and originally was isolated from it, so a direct assessment of its presence can be performed through the examination of chorionic villous samples. Immunofluorescence techniques showed that merosin is strongly expressed in the basement membrane of these villi (Voit et al., 1994). Of course, it is now necessary to check the diagnostic specificity of this approach for a prenatal diagnosis, particularly when the LAMA2 gene defect will be characterized. Prenatal diagnoses have been performed thanks to the detection of merosin in chorionic villous samples, and were controlled at molecular genetics level (Vignier et al., submitted).

The fourth development is about future therapeutic strategies. An animal model of merosin deficiency was detected almost simultaneously by three groups (Arahata et al., 1993; Sunada et al., 1994; Xu et al., 1994). Actually it was a rediscovery of one of the most ancient models of muscular dystrophy, dy/dy mice. We should remember that this model was discarded after the demonstration by Bradley & Jenkinson (1975) of myelination abnormalities in the spinal roots of these mice. As merosin is expressed both in Schwann and muscle basement membranes, this association is now better understood. It should also be remembered that early experiments of muscle cell grafting showed a dramatic improvement of dy^{2j}/dy^{2j} dystrophic mice behaviour (Law et al., 1990). Results of these experiments were strongly discussed. However the extracellular location of the missing protein may allow various strategies to restore its presence at the periphery of the muscle fibres, and perhaps to modify the severely disabling course of these dystrophies.

References

Afifi, A., Zellweger, H., McCormick, W.F. & Mergner, W. (1969): Congenital muscular dystrophy: light and electron microscopic observations. *J. Neurol. Neurosurg. Psychiatry* **32**, 273–280.

Arahata, K., Hayashi, Y.K., Koga, R., Goto, K., Lee, J.H., Miyagoe, Y., Ishii, H., Tsukahara, T., Takeda, S., Woo, M., Nonaka, I., Matsuzaki, T. & Sugita, H. (1993): Laminin in animal models for muscular dystrophy: defect of laminin M in skeletal and cardiac muscles and peripheral nerve of homozygous dystrophic dy/dy mice. *Proc. Jpn Acad.* **69**, Series B, 259–264.

Arikawa, E., Ishihara, T., Nonaka, I., Sugita, H. & Arahata, K. (1991): Immunocytochemical analysis of dystrophin in congenital muscular dystrophy. *J. Neurol. Sci.* **105**, 79–87.

Banker, B.Q. (1994): The congenital muscular dystrophies. In: *Myology*, 2nd edition, eds A.G. Engel & C. Franzini Armstrong, pp. 1275–1289. New York: McGraw-Hill.

Bernier, J.P., Brooke, M., Naidich, R. & Caroll, J. (1979): Myoencephalopathy: cerebral hyomyelination revealed by CT scanner of the head in a muscle disease. *Trans. Am. Neurol. Ass.* **104**, 244–246.

Bradley, W.G. & Jenkinson, M. (1975): Neural abnormalities in dystrophic mouse. *J. Neurol. Sci.* **25**, 249–255.

Burgeson, R.E., Chiquet, M., Deutzmann, R., Ekblom, P., Engel, J., Kleinman, H., Martin, G.R., Meneguzzi, G., Paulsson, M., Sanes, J., Timpl, R., Tryggvason, K., Yamada, Y. & Yurchenco, P.D. (1994): A new nomenclature for the laminins. *Matrix Biol.* **14**, 209–211.

Campbell, K.P. & Kahl, S.D. (1989): Association of dystrophin and an integral membrane glycoprotein. *Nature* **338**, 259–262.

Dobyns, W.B., Pagon, R.A., Armstrong-Curry, C.J.R., Greenberg, F., Grix, A., Holmes, L.B., Laxora, R., Michels, V.V., Robinow, M. & Zimmermann, R.L. (1989): Diagnostic criteria for Walter–Warburg syndrome. *Am. J. Med. Genet.* **32**, 195–210.

Donner, M., Sapola, J. & Somer, H. (1975): Congenital muscular dystrophy: a clinico-pathological and follow up study of 15 patients. *Neuropaediatrie* **6**, 239–258.

Duance, V.C., Stephens, H.R., Dunn, M., Bailey, A.J. & Dubowitz, V. (1980): A role for collagen in the pathogenesis of muscular dystrophy? *Nature* **284**, 470–472.

Dubowitz, V. (1973): Rigid spine syndrome: a muscle syndrome in search of a name. *Proc. R. Soc. Med.* **66**, 219.

Echenne, B., Arthuis, M., Billard, C., Campos-Castello, J., Castel, Y., Dulac, O., Fontan, D., Gauthier, A., Kulakowski, S., De Meuron, G., Moore, J.R., Nieto-Barrera, M., Pages, M., Parain, D., Pavone, L. & Ponsot, G. (1986): Congenital muscular dystrophy and cerebral CT scan anomalies. Results of a collaborative study of the 'Société de Neurologie Infantile'. *J. Neurol. Sci.* **75**, 7–22.

Egger, J., Kendall, B.E., Erdohazi, M., Lake, B.D., Wilson, J. & Brett, E.M. (1983): Involvement of the central nervous system in congenital muscular dystrophies. *Dev. Med. Child. Neurol.* **25**, 32–42.

Ehrig, K., Leivo, I., Scott Agraves, W., Ruoslahti, E. & Engvall, E. (1990): Merosin, a tissue specific basement membrane protein, is a laminin-like protein. *Proc. Natl Acad. Sci. USA* **87**, D 3264–3268.

Engvall, E. (1993): Laminin variants: why, where and when? *Kidney Int.* **43**, 2–6.

Ervasti, J.M. & Campbell, K.P. (1991): Membrane organization of the dystrophin–glycoprotein complex. *Cell* **66**, 1121–1131.

Fardeau, M., Godet-Guillain, J., Tomé, F.M.S., Carson, S. & Whalen, R.G. (1978): Congenital neuromuscular disorders: a critical review. In: *Current topics in nerve and muscle research*, eds A.J. Aguayo & G. Karpati, pp. 164–177. Amsterdam: Excerpta Medica.

Fardeau, M. & Tomé, F.M.S. (1994): Clinical and immunocytochemical evidence of heterogeneity in classical (occidental) congenital muscular dystrophy. In: *Proceedings of the International Symposium on Congenital Muscular Dystrophies*, ed. Y. Fukuyama, Tokyo, 7–8 July 1994 (in press).

Fidzianska, A., Goebel, H.H., Lenard, H.G. & Heckmann, C. (1982): Congenital muscular dystrophy (CMD): a collagen-formative disease? *J. Neurol. Sci.* **55**, 79–90.

Fukuyama, Y., Kawazura, M. & Haruna, H. (1960): A peculiar form of congenital progressive muscular dystrophy – report of fifteen cases. *Pediatr. Univ. Tokyo* **4**, 5–8.

Fukuyama, Y., Osawa, M. & Suzuki, H. (1981): Congenital progressive muscular dystrophy of the Fukuyama type – clinical, genetic and pathological considerations. *Brain Dev.* **3**, 1–29.

Hantaï, D., Labat-Robert, J., Grimaud, J.A. & Fardeau, M. (1985): Fibronectin, laminin, type I, II, III and IV collagen in Duchenne's muscular dystrophy, congenital muscular dystrophies and congenital myopathies: an immunocytochemical study. *Connect. Tissue Res.* **13**, 273–281.

Hayashi, Y.K., Engvall, E., Arikawa-Hirasawa, E., Goto, K., Koga, R., Nonaka, I., Sugita, H. & Arahata, K. (1993): Abnormal localization of laminin subunits in muscular dystrophies. *J. Neurol. Sci.* **119**, 53–64.

Helbling-Leclerc, A., Topaloglu, H., Tomé, F., Sewry, C., Gyapay, G., Weissenbach, J., Muntoni, F., Schwartz, K., Fardeau, M., Guicheney, P. (1995): Readjusting the localization of laminin a2-chain deficiency CMD locus on chromosome 6q2. *C. R. Acad. Sci. Paris* **318**, 1245–1252.

Helbling-Leclerc, A., Zhang, X., Topaloglu, H., Cruaud, C., Tesson, F., Weissenbach, J., Tomé, F., Schwartz, K., Fardeau, M., Tryggvason, K., Guicheney, P. (1995): Mutations in the laminin a2-chain gene (LAMA2) cause merosin-deficient congenital dystrophy. *Nature Genetics* **11**, 216–218.

Hillaire, D., Leclerc, A., Faure, S., Topaloglu, H., Chiannilkulchai, N., Guicheney, P., Grinas, L., Legos, P., Philpot, J., Evangelista, T., Routon, M.C., Mayer, M., Pellissier, J.F., Estournet, B., Barois, A., Hentati, F., Feingold, N., Beckmann, J.S., Dubowitz, V., Tomé, F.M.S. & Fardeau, M. (1994): Localization of merosin-negative congenital muscular dystrophy to chromosome 6q2 by homozygosity mapping. *Hum. Mol. Genet.* **3**, 1657–1661.

Howard, R. (1908): A case of congenital defect of the muscular system (dystrophia muscularis congenita) and its association with congenital talipes equino-varus. *Proc. R. Soc. Med.* **1**, 157–166.

Ibraghimov-Beskrovnaya, O., Ervasti, J.M., Leveille, C.J., Slaughter, C.A., Sernett, S.W. & Campbell, K.P. (1992): Primary structure of dystrophin-associated glycoproteins linking dystrophin to extracellular matrix. *Nature* **355**, 696–702.

Law, P.K., Goudwin, T.G., Li, H.J., Ajamoughli, G. & Chen, M. (1990): Myoblast transfer improves muscle genetics structure function and normalizes the behavior and life-span of dystrophic mice. *Adv. Exp. Med. Biol.* **280**, 75–87.

Leivo, I. & Engvall, E. (1988): Merosine, a protein specific for basement membrane of Schwann cells, striated muscle, and trophoblast, is expressed late in nerve and muscle development. *Proc. Natl Acad. Sci. USA* **85**, 1544–1548.

Lichtig, C., Ludatscher, R.M., Mandel, H. & Gershoni-Baruch, R. (1993): Muscle involvement in Walker–Warburg syndrome. Clinicopathologic features of four cases. *Am. J. Clin. Pathol.* **100**, 493–496.

Nissinen, M., Helbling-Leclerc, A., Zhang, X., Evangelista, T., Topaloglu, H., Cruaud, C., Weissenbach, J., Schwartz, K., Fardeau, M., Tomé, F., Tryggvason, K., Guicheney, P. (1996): Substitution of a conserved cysteine-996 in a cysteine-rich motif of the laminin a-2 chain in congenital muscular dystrophy. *Am. J. Hum. Genet.* **58**, 1177–1184.

Nonaka, I. & Chou, S. (1979): Congenital muscular dystrophy. In: *Handbook of clinical neurology*, Vol. **41**, eds P.J. Winken & G.W. Bruyn, pp. 27–50. Amsterdam: North-Holland Publishing Company.

Osawa, M. (1978): A genetical and epidemiological study on congenital progressive muscular dystrophy (Fukuyama type). *J. Tokyo Women's Med. Coll.* (Tokyo) **8**, 112–149.

Osawa, M., Arai, Y., Ikenaka, H., Murasugi, H., Suguhara, N., Sumida, S., Okada, N., Shishikura, K., Suzuki, H., Hirayama, Y., Hirasawa, K., Fukuyama, Y., Tsutsumi, A., Ito, K. & Uchida, Y. (1991): Fukuyama type congenital progressive muscular dystrophy. *Acta Paediatr. Jpn* **33**, 261–269.

Pavone, L., Gullotta, F., Grasso, S. & Vanucchi, C. (1986): Hydrocephalus lissencephaly, ocular abnormalities and congenital muscular dystrophy. A Warburg syndrome variant? *Neuropediatrics* **17**, 206–211.

Philpot, J., Sewry, C., Pennock, J. & Dubowitz, V. (1995): Clinical phenotype in congenital muscular dystrophy: correlation with expression of merosin in skeletal muscle. *Neuromusc. Disord.* **5**, 301–305.

Santavuori, P., Leisti, J. & Kruus, J. (1977): Muscle, eye and brain disease: a new syndrome. *Neuropaediatrie* **8**, 550–553.

Serratrice, G., Cros, D., Pellissier, J.F., Gastaut, J.L. & Pouget, J. (1980): Dystrophie musculaire congénitale. *Rev. Neurol. (Paris)* **136**, 445–472.

Sunada, Y., Bernier, S.M., Kozak, C.A., Yamada, Y. & Campbell, K.P. (1994): Deficiency of merosin in dystrophic dy mice and genetic linkage of the laminin M chain gene to dy locus. *J. Biol. Chem.* **269**, 13729–13732.

Toda, T., Segawa, M., Nomura, Y., Nonaka, I., Masuda, K., Ishihara, T., Suzuki, M., Tomita, I., Uriguchi, Y., Ohno, K., Misugi, M., Sasaki, Y., Takada, K., Kawai, M., Otani, K., Murakami, T., Saito, K., Fukuyama, Y., Shimizu, T., Kanazawa, I. & Nakamura, Y. (1993): Localization of a gene for Fukuyama type congenital muscular dystrophy to chromosome 9q31–33. *Nature Genet.* **5**, 283–286.

Tomé, F.M.S., Evangelista, T., Leclerc, A., Sunada, Y., Manole, E., Estournet, B., Barois, A., Campbell, K.P. & Fardeau, M. (1994): Congenital muscular dystrophy with merosin deficiency. *C. R. Acad. Sci. Paris* **317**, 351–357.

Topaloglu, H., Evangelista, T., Gögüs, S., Yalaz, K. & Tomé, F.M.S. (1994): Merosin and clinical characteristics of congenital muscular dystrophy in an unselected group of Turkish patients. *Brain Dev.* (in press).

Trevisan, C., Carollo, C.P., Segalla, P., Angelini, C., Drigo, P. & Giordano, R. (1991): Congenital muscular dystrophy: brain alterations in an unselected series of Western patients. *J. Neurol. Neurosurg. Psychiatry* **54**, 330–334.

Trevisan, C.P., Martinello, F., Ferruzza, E. & Angelini, C. (1995): Divergence of central nervous system involvement in two western sisters with congenital muscular dystrophy. *Eur. Neurol.* (in press).

Ullrich O. (1930): Kongenitale, atonisch-sclerotische Muskeldystrophie, ein weiterer Typus der heredodegenerativen Erkränkungen des neuromusculären Systems. *Z. Ges. Neurol. Psychiat.* **126**, 171–201.

Vignier, N., Helbling-Leclerc, A., Zhang, X., Paquis, V., Richelme, C., Cruaud, C., Chevallay, M., Lambert, J.C. Schwartz, K., Fardeau, M., Tryggvason, K., Tomé, F.M.S., Guicheney, P. (submitted): Detection of a cytosine deletion in exon 16 of the laminin a2-chain gene (LAMA2) at position 2418: prenatal exclusion in a fetus at risk of congenital muscular dystrophy with laminin a2-chain deficiency.

Voit, T., Fardeau, M. & Tomé, F.M.S. (1994): Prenatal detection of merosin expression in human placenta. *Neuropediatrics* **25**, 332–333.

Vuolteenaho, R., Nissinen, M., Sainio, K., Byers, M., Eddy, R., Hirvonen H., Shows T.B., Sariola, H., Engvall, E. & Tryggvason, K. (1994): Human laminin M chain (merosin): complete primary structure, chromosomal assignment, and expression of the M and A chain in human fetal tissues. *J. Cell Biol.* **124**, 381–394.

Xu H., Christmas, P., Wu, X.R., Wever, U.M. & Engvall, E. (1994): Defective muscle basement membrane and lack of M-laminin in the dystrophic *dy/dy* mouse. *Proc. Natl. Acad. Sci. USA* **91**, 5572–5576.

Zellweger, H., Afifi, A., McCormick, W.F. & Mergner, W. (1967a): Benign congenital muscular dystrophy. A special form of congenital hypotonia. *Clin. Pediatr.* **6**, 655–663.

Zellweger, H., Afifi, A., McCormick, W.F. & Mergner, W. (1967b): Severe congenital muscular dystrophy. *Am. J. Dis. Child.* **114**, 591–602.

Chapter 4

Dystrophinopathies

Lucia Morandi, Marina Mora, Claudia Di Blasi, Rita Barresi and Valeria Confalonieri

Department of Neuromuscular Diseases, National Neurological Institute 'Carlo Besta', Via Celoria 11, 20133 Milan, Italy

Summary

Duchenne's and Becker's muscular dystrophies are the most common X-linked diseases caused by mutations of the dystrophin gene. Duchenne's muscular dystrophy (DMD) is the more severe condition leading to loss of autonomous walking early in childhood and death in the second decade due to respiratory insufficiency. Becker muscular dystrophy (BMD) is characterized by a later age of onset and milder progression. In both disorders, muscle involvement has a similar distribution although cardiomyopathy is more common in BMD patients. The site and the extent of the gene deletions are common to both diseases. Maintenance of the reading frame, allowing synthesis of a qualitatively altered and partially functional dystrophin, is responsible for the less severe clinical phenotype of BMD. Thus, immunochemical analysis of dystrophin expression in muscle is the only reliable modality for distinguishing the two conditions in infancy. In addition to DMD and BMD, several other clinical phenotypes with molecular defects in the gene and dystrophin abnormalities, have been delineated. Moreover, altered dystrophin expression has been reported in asymptomatic and symptomatic DMD and BMD carriers.

Introduction

Since the characterization of the Duchenne's muscular dystrophy gene and its protein product dystrophin, numerous patients have been reported with molecular defects in the gene and abnormalities in dystrophin (Ahn & Kunkel, 1993). These patients present a considerable range of clinical phenotypes and thus a broad spectrum of dystrophinopathies has been delineated. The most common phenotypes are the Duchenne's (DMD) and Becker's (BMD) muscular dystrophies; the clinical progression of DMD varies somewhat while that of BMD is highly variable.

Duchenne's muscular dystrophy

DMD is the most severe muscular dystrophy. The first symptoms – difficulty in running, jumping and climbing stairs – are observed early in childhood and are due to weakness of the pelvic and lower limb muscles. This weakness, often associated with early muscle contractures and tendon retractions, spreads progressively to the upper limbs and to the paravertebral muscles where it produces scoliosis and increased lumbar lordosis. Walking becomes progressively more difficult, and independent gait is lost at about 9 years of age. DMD patients die in their twenties due to respiratory insufficiency. Dystrophin is completely or almost completely absent from the muscles of DMD patients, and is already absent in affected foetuses. No patients lacking dystrophin have ever been reported with a clinical phenotype other than DMD. The invariable relationship between dystrophin absence and the DMD phenotype is due to a deletion in the gene that disrupts the reading frame resulting in incompletely translated mRNA and altered dystrophin molecules that cannot be normally integrated into the membrane and are catabolized very rapidly. However, in about two-thirds of DMD patients a few muscle fibres with weak dystrophin-positive immunolabelling can be detected using antibodies raised against fragments of the dystrophin molecule. Such fragments may come from after as well as before the point corresponding to the frame-shifting deletion in the dystrophin gene. By immunoblot techniques, a faint dystrophin band of normal or near-normal molecular weight can often be detected in muscles. Weakly dystrophin-positive fibres apparently occur more frequently in patients with deletion of exon 44 or exon 45. In such cases the presence of dystrophin is probably due to restoration of the reading frame at the level of RNA transcripts – this may occur by skipping one or two exons adjacent to the original mutation. A correlation between the abundance of these in-frame mRNA transcripts and the abundance of dystrophin has been reported by Nicholson (1993). The clinical phenotype of DMD patients with no detectable dystrophin is more severe than in those with low levels: the mean age at loss of independent walking correlates with the quantity of dystrophin present as determined by densitometric analysis. Loss of walking may be posponed to 11–13 years in cases of dystrophin abundance which is 25 per cent of normal (Nicholson, 1993).

Mental retardation occurs frequently in DMD patients (but rarely in BMD patients). A dystrophin isoform very similar to muscle dystrophin is expressed in the brain and is controlled by a different promoter (the cortical promoter) (Nudel et al., 1989; Barnea et al., 1990). In addition, three other promoters have been detected recently; these regulate dystrophin translation in non-muscle tissues, including the brain (Tubiello et al., 1995). However, analysis of the brain-specific cortical promoter region in DMD and BMD patients failed to detect mutations (den Dunnen et al., 1991; Tubiello et al., 1995). Furthermore, Rapaport et al. (1992) have reported a DMD patient with normal mental function having a deletion in the cortical promoter extending into the first 18 exons of the dystrophin gene. Mechanisms in addition to the absence of dystrophin are therefore likely to be responsible for the intellectual impairment found in a significant proportion of DMD patients. Intellectual impairment has been reported associated with deletions encompassing exon 52 in several patients (Rapaport et al., 1991).

Recently a 6.5 kb mRNA transcribed from the dystrophin gene has been found. This transcript codes for a 70.8 kD protein containing only the C-terminal and cysteine-rich domains of dystrophin; it is probably transcribed from a different promoter and is a major product of the dystrophin gene in the brain, neuronal and glial cell cultures, and many non-muscle tissues (Bar et al., 1990; Lederfein et al., 1992). Absence or dysfunction of the protein encoded by this mRNA may be involved in DMD-associated mental impairment.

Becker's muscular dystrophy

Becker muscular dystrophy is the other allelic disease of the DMD locus. In both dystrophies, deletions occur at the same sites and may have the same extension; the less severe clinical phenotype of BMD is due to maintenance of the reading frame (Monaco et al., 1988; Koenig et al., 1989) which allows synthesis of a smaller dystrophin molecule, or one with altered amino acid sequence, that retains some functionality (Hoffman et al., 1988). Dystrophin is anchored to the sarcolemma through a glycoprotein complex which binds to the cysteine-rich and C-terminal domains (Ervasti & Campbell, 1991); these domains are always retained in the dystrophin protein in BMD (Arahata et al., 1991; Morandi et al., 1995).

There is considerable variability of phenotype among BMD patients, often among those in the same family. Maps of correlations between clinical symptoms, gene deletions and consequent domain abnormalities have been proposed by several authors (Bushby *et al.*, 1993a; Angelini *et al.*, 1994; Comi *et al.*, 1994).

We investigated this variability in a study carried out in our laboratory which compared dystrophin expression in muscles with clinical phenotype. We investigated dystrophin expression immuno-chemically by means of six antibodies raised against six different regions of dystrophin (Morandi *et al.*, 1995). Our BMD patients showed two distinct patterns of dystrophin expression. In group A (29 patients) we observed the typical patchy distribution of dystrophin on muscle fibres (indicating variable protein expression on the sarcolemma of a single muscle fibre and from one fibre to another); the protein itself was of normal or slightly reduced molecular weight by Western blot (but two patients in this group had dystrophin of increased molecular weight due to duplication within the gene). By contrast, the 30 group B patients lacked or had reduced expression of dystrophin, according to only one of our antibodies (implying lack or alteration of a restricted portion of the dystrophin molecule, with variable alteration of an adjacent portion in a few cases), but normal or near normal dystrophin expression according to the remaining five antibodies against other portions of the protein. By immunoblot, the protein band was absent or of reduced intensity using the antibody against the altered portion; but a band of variably reduced molecular weight was detected with the other antibodies.

Before the age of 10, the clinical phenotype was very mild in both these groups of patients, but from 11 to 30 years disease progression differed substantially, with a milder clinical picture in group B. The molecular weight of dystrophin was normal or slightly reduced in group A and was variably reduced, generally conspicuously so, in group B. The amount of dystrophin expressed varied markedly in both groups. The pattern of immunohistochemical staining in group B patients correlated with a milder clinical phenotype, suggesting that small dystrophin molecules lacking a portion in the N-terminus or in the rod domain, are more functional than proteins with normal or slightly reduced molecular weight that display the typical patchy distribution at the sarcolemma.

None of our BMD patients lacked the D10 portion of the dystrophin protein that is localized in the cystein-rich domain, close to the C-terminus; this finding is indicative of the fact that these regions are concerned with linking dystrophin to the glycoprotein complex and stabilizing the membrane (Ervasti & Campbell, 1991).

We analysed densitometrically the dystrophin in our BMD patients' muscles and found that the quantity of dystrophin present varied from patient to patient, with no obvious relationship between dystrophin abundance and clinical stage or immunohistochemical results. Other authors have sought to relate dystrophin abundance to clinical phenotype and disease progression (Bushby *et al.*, 1993a; Comi *et al.*, 1994; Angelini *et al.*, 1994); some correlation between increasing dystrophin abundance and milder clinical course was reported, but the detailed conclusions of these studies differed markedly.

Unusual forms of dystrophinopathy

Cases of dystrophinopathy presenting as congenital muscular dystrophy have been described by Prelle and by Kiriakides. The first case, a 5-year-old boy, presented as a floppy infant with early delay in motor development and mental retardation (Prelle *et al.*, 1992). The second, a 3.5-year-old boy, had congenital hypotonia, calf pseudohypertrophy, delayed motor milestones and joint contractures (Kiriakides *et al.*, 1994). Both had very high plasma CK levels, dystrophic features in muscle biopsy and no dystrophin.

Gospe *et al.* (1989) reported an atypical BMD phenotype in a family presenting only cramps and myalgia. Several of our patients (in both groups of the study described above) had myalgia, and five of the six patients with an abnormality in the 30 kD portion of the molecule suffered myalgia associated with various degrees of weakness. Sunohara *et al.* (1990) reported four patients with a slowly progressive weakness initially confined to the quadriceps muscles, with faint and discontinuous patchy dystrophin expression on immunostaining and a protein band of reduced intensity and molecular weight on immunoblot. Quadriceps myopathy is a rather heterogeneous disorder: inflammatory myopathies, spinal muscular atrophies, and ill-defined forms of limb girdle muscular dystrophy can all produce a quadriceps myopathy. It is now clear that patients with this phenotype should have muscle biopsies and be analysed immunochemically for dystrophin because they may be unusual presentations of BMD.

A unique case of dystrophinopathy was reported recently (Dworzak *et al.*, 1994) in a male infant presenting bilateral diaphragm paralysis, muscle weakness, ptosis of the eyelids, facial dysmorphisms and bilateral cryptorchidism at birth. The CK level was normal, as was EMG. A muscle biopsy showed type II hypertrophy. Dystrophin was almost negative to anti-D8 antibody and had a patchy distribution with the six other antibodies used. Deletion of exons 49–53 was detected by DNA analysis.

DMD and BMD carriers

Abnormal expression of dystrophin has been found in the muscles of DMD and BMD carriers (Arahata *et al.*, 1989; Bonilla *et al.*, 1988; Hoffman *et al.*, 1992). Dystrophin may be totally or partially absent from the sarcolemma of a proportion of muscle fibres in DMD carriers, while in BMD carriers it may have a patchy distribution (Haginoya *et al.*, 1991; Bushby *et al.*, 1993b). We have analysed a series of DMD and BMD carriers using the panel of six antibodies against the dystrophin molecule mentioned above (Morandi *et al.*, 1995). We were able to identify BMD carriers having a mosaic pattern of dystrophin expression detected only with one antibody (Mora *et al.*, 1993). This is in agreement with our observations in BMD patients which revealed the absence of restricted portions of the protein only. Mosaicism was observed only in carriers with increased CK levels (Morandi *et al.*, 1990), both in patients with mild clinical signs and in asymptomatic women. Symptomatic carriers usually present larger numbers of dystrophin-negative fibres than asymptomatic women. The percentage of mosaic fibres present has been reported to be age related, being higher in young girls (Hoffman *et al.*, 1992), but this is controversial.

In the diagnostic work-up of females with high plasma CK, a family history of dystrophinopathy and clinical symptoms, the expression of muscle dystrophin should always be evaluated. Normal dystrophin does not exclude the carrier condition however and for appropriate genetic counselling a DNA analysis (by RFLPs) of the female, the proband and family members is necessary.

Some myopathic females with mosaicism have been reported with dystrophinopathy secondary to X-autosome translocation; such myopathies can be identified by performing a karyotype.

Cardiac involvement in dystrophinopathy

Altered dystrophin expression in myocytes may cause cardiac involvement in both DMD and BMD. The affected patients present a reduction in cardiac contractility or a variable increase in left ventricular diameter, or both. Cardiomyopathy may be the first symptom in BMD patients. Among 29 of our BMD patients who underwent cardiac ultrasonography, eight showed variable degrees of cardiac involvement. We found no specific correlations between cardiac abnormalities and dystrophin expression or deletions in the dystrophin gene, as previously reported by others (Koenig *et al.*, 1989; Bushby *et al.*, 1993a). Two of our patients had severe cardiomyopathy. One received a cardiac transplant at age 22, his skeletal muscle lacked the D8 portion of dystrophin and exons 45–52 were deleted; he was moderately affected when last seen at the age of 30. In the other, dystrophin expression was patchy with all antibodies by immunohistochemistry and of increased molecular weight by Western blot. He had severe muscle weakness. A similar type of cardiac involvement has been described in a few DMD carriers (Sewry et al., 1993).

References

Ahn, A.H. & Kunkel, L.M. (1993): The structural and functional diversity of dystrophin. *Nature Genet.* **3**, 283–291.

Angelini, C., Fanin, M., Pegoraro, E., Freda, M.P., Cadaldini, M. & Martinello, F. (1994): Clinical-molecular correlations in 104 mild X-linked muscular dystrophy patients: characterization of sub-clinical phenotypes. *Neuromusc. Disord.* **4**, 349–358.

Arahata, K., Ishihara, T., Kamakura, K., Tsukahara, T., Ishiura, S., Baba, C., Matsumoto, T., Nonaka, I. & Sugita, H. (1989): Mosaic expression of dystrophin in symptomatic carriers of Duchenne's muscular dystrophy. *N. Engl. J. Med.* **320**, 138–142.

Arahata, K., Beggs, A.H., Honda, H., Ito, S., Ishiura, S., Tsukahara, T., Ishiguro, T., Eguchi, C., Orimo, S., Arikawa, E., Kaido, M., Nonaka, I., Sugita, H. & Kunkel, L.M. (1991): Preservation of the C-terminus of dystrophin molecule in the skeletal muscle from Becker muscular dystrophy. *J. Neurol. Sci.* **101**, 148–156.

Bar, S., Barnea, E., Levy, Z., Neuman, S., Yaffe, D. & Nudel, U. (1990): A novel product of the DMD gene which greatly differs from the known isoforms in its structure and tissue distribution. *Biochem. J.* **272**, 557–560.

Barnea, E., Zuk, D., Simantov, R., Nudel, U. & Yaffe, D. (1990): Specificity of expression of the muscle and brain dystrophin gene promoters in muscle and brain cells. *Neuron* **5**, 881–888.

Bonilla, E., Schmidt, B., Samitt, C.E., Miranda, A.F., Hays, A.P., De Oliveira, A.B.S., Chang, H.W., Servidei, S., Ricci, E., Younger, D.S. & Di Mauro, S. (1988): Normal and dystrophin-deficient muscle fibers in carriers of the gene for Duchenne muscular dystrophy. *Am. J. Pathol.* **133**, 440–445.

Bushby, K.M.D., Gardner-Medwin, D., Nicholson, L.V.B., Johnson, M.A., Haggerty, I.D., Cleghorn, M.J., Harris, J.B. & Bhattacharya, S.S. (1993a): The clinical, genetic and dystrophin characteristics of Becker muscular dystrophy. II. Correlation of phenotype with genetic and protein abnormalities. *J. Neurol.* **240**, 105–112.

Bushby, K.M.D., Goodship, J.A., Nicholson, L.V.B., Johnson, M.A., Haggerty, I.D. & Gardner-Medwin, D. (1993b): Variability in clinical, genetic and protein abnormalities in manifesting carriers of Duchenne and Becker muscular dystrophy. *Neuromusc. Disord.* **3**, 57–64.

Comi, G.P., Prelle, A., Bresolin, N., Moggio, M., Bardoni, A., Gallanti, A., Vita, G., Toscano, A., Ferro, M.T., Bordoni, A., Fortunato, S., Ciscato, P., Felisari, G., Tedeschi, S., Castelli, E., Garghentino, R., Turconi, A., Fraschini, P., Marchi, E., Negretto, G.G., Adobbati, L., Meola, G., Tonin, P., Papadimitriou, A. & Scarlato, G. (1994): Clinical variability in Becker muscular dystrophy. Genetic, biochemical and immunohistochemical correlates. *Brain* **117**, 1–14.

den Dunnen, J.T., Casula, L., Makover, A., Bakker, B., Yaffe, D., Nudel, U. & van Ommen, G.J.B. (1991): Mapping of dystrophin brain promoter: a deletion of this region is compatible with normal intellect. *Neuromusc. Disord.* **5**, 327–331.

Dworzak, F., Mora, M., Morandi, L., Bernasconi, P. & Cornelio, F. (1994): A unique case of dystrophinopathy. *J. Neurol. Neurosurg. Psychiatry* **57**, 1136–1147.

Ervasti, J.M. & Campbell, K.P. (1991): Membrane organization of the dystrophin-glycoprotein complex. *Cell* **66**, 1121–1131.

Gospe, S.M. Jr., Lazaro, R.P., Lava, N.S., Grootscholten, P.M., Scott, M.O. & Fischbeck, K.H. (1989): Familial X-linked myalgia and cramps: a nonprogressive myopathy associated with a deletion in the dystrophin gene. *Neurology* **39**, 1277–1280.

Haginoya, K., Yamamoto, K., Iinuma, K., Yanagisawa, T., Ichinohasama, Y., Shimmoto, M., Suzuki, Y. & Tada, K. (1991): Dystrophin immunohistochemistry in a symptomatic carrier of Becker muscular dystrophy. *J. Neurol.* **238**, 375–378.

Hoffman, E.P., Fischbeck, K.H., Brown, R.H., Johnson, M., Medori, R., Loike, J.D., Harris, J.B., Waterston, R., Brooke, M., Specht, L., Kupsky, W., Chamberlain, J., Caskey, T., Shaphiro, F. & Kunkel, L.M. (1988): Characterization of dystrophin in muscle-biopsies specimens from patients with Duchenne's or Becker's muscular dystrophy. *N. Engl. J. Med.* **318**, 1363–1368.

Hoffman, E.P., Arahata, K., Minetti, C., Bonilla, E. Rowland, L.P. *et al.* (1992): Dystrophinopathy in isolated cases of myopathy in females. *Neurology* **42**, 967–975.

Koenig, M., Beggs, A.H., Moyer, M., Scherpf, S., Heindrichs, K., Bettecken, T., Meng, G., Muller, C.R., Lindlof, M., Kaariainen, H., de la Chapelle, A., Kiuru, A., Savontaus, M-L., Gilgenkrantz, H., Recan, D., Chelly, J., Kaplan, J-C., Covone, A.E., Archidiacono, N., Romeo, G., Liechti-Gallati, S., Schneider, V., Braga, S., Moser, H., Darras, B.T., Murphy, P., Francke, U., Chen, J.D., Morgan, G., Denton, M., Greenberg, C.R., Wrogemann, K., Blonden, L.A.J., van Paassen, H.M.B., van Ommen, G.J.B. & Kunkel, L.M. (1989): The molecular basis for Duchenne versus Becker molecular dystrophy: correlation of severity with type of deletion. *Am. J. Hum. Genet.* **45**, 498–506.

Kiriakides, T., Gabriel, G., Drousiotou, A., Meznanic-Petrusa, M. & Middleton, L. (1994): Dystrophinopathy presenting as congenital muscular dystrophy. *Neuromusc. Disord.* **4**, 387–392.

Lederfein, D., Levy, Z., Augier, N., Mornet, D., Morris, G., Fuchs, O., Yaffe, D. & Nudel, U. (1992): A 71 kDa protein is a major product of the Duchenne muscular dystrophy gene in brain and other nonmuscle tissues. *Proc. Natl. Acad. Sci. USA* **89**, 5346–5350.

Monaco, A.P., Bertelson, C.J., Liechti-Gallati, S., Moser, H. & Kunkel, L.M. (1988): An explanation for the phenotypic differences between patients bearing partial deletions of the DMD locus. *Genomics* **2**, 90–95.

Mora, M., Morandi, L., Piccinelli, A., Gussoni, E., Gebbia, M., Blasevich, F., Dworzak, F. & Cornelio, F. (1993): Dystrophin abnormalities in Duchenne and Becker dystrophy carriers: correlation with cytoskeletal proteins and myosins. *J. Neurol.* **240**, 455–461.

Morandi, L., Mora, M., Gussoni, E., Tedeschi, S. & Cornelio, F. (1990): Dystrophin analysis in Duchenne and Becker muscular dystrophy carriers: correlation with intracellular calcium and albumin. *Ann. Neurol.* **28**, 674–679.

Morandi, L., Mora, M., Confalonieri, V., Barresi, R., Di Blasi, C., Brugnoni, R., Bernasconi, P., Mantegazza, R., Dworzak, F., Antozzi, C., Balestrini, M.R., Jarre, L., Pini, A., Merlini, R., Piccolo, G., Mazzanti, A., Daniel, S., Blasevich, F. & Cornelio, F. (1995): Dystrophin characterization in BMD patients: correlation of abnormal protein with clinical phenotype. *J. Neurol. Sci.* **132**, 146–155.

Nicholson, L.V.B. (1993): The 'rescue' of dystrophin synthesis in boys with Duchenne muscular dystrophy. *Neuromusc. Disord.* **3**, 525–531.

Nudel, U., Zuk, D., Einat, P., Zeelon, E., Levy, Z., Neuman, S. & Yaffe, D. (1989): Duchenne muscular dystrophy gene product is not identical in muscle and brain. *Nature* **337**, 76–78.

Prelle, A., Medori, R., Moggio, M., Chan, H.W., Gallanti, A., Scarlato, G. & Bonilla, E. (1992): Dystrophin deficiency in a case of congenital myopathy. *J. Neurol.* **239**, 76–78.

Rapaport, D., Passos-Bueno, M.R., Brandao, L., Love, D., Vainzof, M. & Zatz, M. (1991): Apparent association of mental retardation and specific patterns of deletions screened with probes cf56a and cf23a in Duchenne muscular dystrophy. *Am. J. Med. Genet.* **39**, 437–441.

Rapaport, D., Passos-Bueno, M.R., Takata, R.I., Campiotto, S., Eggers, S., Vainzof, M., Makover, A., Nudel, U., Yaffe, D. & Zatz, M. (1992): A deletion including the brain promoter of the Duchenne muscular dystrophy gene is not associated with mental retardation. *Neuromusc. Disord.* **2**, 117–120.

Sewry, C.A., Sansone, A., Clerk, A., Sherratt, T.G., Hasson, N., Rodillo, E., Heckmatt, J.Z., Strong, P.N. & Dubowitz, V. (1993): Manifesting carriers of Xp21 muscular dystrophy: lack of correlation between dystrophin expression and clinical weakness. *Neuromusc. Disord.* **3**, 141–148.

Sunohara, N., Arahata, K., Hoffman, E.P., Yamada, H., Nishimiya, J., Arikawa, E., Kaido, M., Nonaka, I. & Sugita, H. (1990): Quadriceps myopathy: forme fruste of Becker muscular dystrophy. *Ann. Neurol.* **28**, 634–639.

Tubiello, G., Carrera, P., Soriani, N., Morandi, L. & Ferrari, M. (1995): Mutational analysis of muscle and brain specific promoter regions of distrophin gene in DMD/BMD Italian patients by denaturing gradient gel electrophoresis (DGGE). *Molec. Cell. Probes* **9**, 441–446.

Chapter 5

The congenital myopathies

Carlo P. Trevisan

Institute of Neurology, University of Padua, Via Giustiniani 5, 35128 Padua, Italy

Summary

A review of the literature on congenital myopathies does not reveal a uniform classification of these neuromuscular disorders: in any case, among them are essentially considered the genetic diseases with structural changes in the skeletal muscle. Several forms have been identified: the most frequently observed are the multiform entity defined as myotubular/centronuclear myopathy, nemaline myopathy and central core disease. In these myopathies, other than characteristic structural changes, a type I fibre predominance is often detected – an aspecific feature that in some floppy infants appears as the only histochemical abnormalitiy. On clinical grounds, these diseases usually present with a variable floppy infant syndrome, even if a late onset is not uncommon. The muscular involvement may range from severe degrees, as in the X-linked variant of myotubular/centronuclear myopathy, to very mild ones, as in central core disease. Skeletal deformities are often associated. The clinical course, usually benign in central core disease, may be various in the other forms, with frequent early fatality in the X-linked variant of myotubular/centronuclear myopathy. Serum CK and EMG findings are of no help in the diagnosis, which can be made only by morphological, histochemical or electron-microscopic evidence of the specific structural changes at muscle biopsy. Recent investigations of immunohistochemistry in muscles of patients with congenital myopathies have allowed a better insight into this still unclear group of diseases, mainly by data on altered cytoskeleton proteins in myotubular/centronuclear myopathy. Ongoing molecular genetic studies have already mapped central core disease to chromosome 19q13.1, X-linked myotubular/centronuclear myopathy to chromosome Xq28, and nemaline myopathy to chromosome 1q21–23 (dominant) and to chromosome 2q21–22 (recessive). Apart from diseases with structural changes in muscle, congenital myopathies should also include the myopathies of metabolic or dystrophic type with neonatal onset. Among them, congenital muscular dystrophy has been the object of recent major immunochemical and genetic studies, which have identified a subtype of the disease with merosin deficiency mapping, which maps to chromosome 6q22–23.

Among the neuromuscular disorders possibly underlying the floppy infant syndrome, congenital myopathies are of major relevance. Before the introduction of histochemical investigations of muscle biopsies in the 1950s, these undiagnosed myopathies were mainly confused into the so-called 'benign congenital hypotonia', a term under which Walton in 1956 grouped all the heterogeneous and undefined forms of infantile hypotonia with a benign clinical course and no detectable muscular alterations. Walton, however, anticipated that the introduction of more sophisticated morphological and biochemical analysis of muscle biopsies would gradually reduce the range of this obscure and uncertain nosographic entity. Actually, in the same year (1956), Shy and Magee identified the first case of central core disease.

Amongst the heterogeneous group of congenital myopathies should be considered all the muscular diseases characterized by muscular pathology of structural, histochemical, metabolic, or dystrophic types evident at birth (Bodensteiner, 1994; Gardner-Medwin, 1994). However, the term congenital myopathies is currently restricted to those with specific structural alterations in skeletal muscle, including changes in the histochemical mosaic (Dubowitz, 1989; Fardeau & Tomé, 1994; Gardner-Medwin, 1994). Generally these myopathies are genetically determined, even if with different individual modes of inheritance (Table 1).

Their usual clinical presentation is that of a non-specific floppy infant syndrome of varying severity; none the less, in some instances they may show clinical evidence of muscular involvement later in childhood or even in adult life. Congenital myopathies with structural changes are considered to be rare diseases, but epidemiological data about them are not available. Moreover, it has to be considered that many of them may easily remain undiagnosed in the neonatal period, if the muscle biopsy is not adequately evaluated by histochemistry and electron microscopy. In our experience, altogether they could be as frequent as Werdnig–Hoffmann disease and congenital muscular dystrophy (Mostacciuolo et al., 1996). In Table 1, classification of congenital myopathies with their possible means of inheritance is shown, together with a brief review of the main characteristics of the most frequent types diagnosed at our Neuromuscular Center.

Table 1. Classification of congenital myopathies

A. Congenital myopathies with structural changes

The major types	Inheritance	The anecdotal types
Centronuclear/ myotubular myopathy	Aut. recessive or dominant; X-linked	Finger print body myopathy
Nemaline myopathy	Aut. dominant or recessive	Reducing body myopathy
Central core disease	Aut. dominant	Zebra body myopathy
Minicore disease	Aut. recessive or dominant	Sarcotubular myopathy
Congenital type 1 fiber predominance	Aut. recessive	Spheroid body myopathy
Congenital fiber type disproportion	Aut. recessive or dominant	Trilaminar aggregates myopathy
		Others

B. Congenital myopathies of dystrophic type

Congenital muscular dystrophy
Congenital myotonic dystrophy

C. Other congenital myopathies

Myotubular/centronuclear myopathy (M/CM)

In our experience, this heterogeneous congenital myopathy is the most frequently diagnosed in a neuromuscular centre, even if nemaline myopathy seems to be the most frequently reported. It was first described in 1966 by Spiro et al. as a myopathy characterized by a congenital and slowly progressive muscular deficit, associated with frequent internal nuclei in muscle fibres. The presence of internal nuclei in more than 25 per cent of the muscle fibres (see Fig. 1) is still considered, at morphological level, to be the essential feature of this myopathy (Wallgren-Pettersson, 1994). In addition, histochemical studies frequently show a perinuclear halo devoid of ATPase activity. The similarity of these characteristics with those of myotubes suggested to the authors the term myotubular myopathy. However, in subsequent reports, the relationship between alterations of this myopathy and the myotubule characteristics was questioned and the term centronuclear myopathy was preferred (Fardeau & Tomé, 1994; Gardner-Medwin, 1994) to indicate this heterogeneous nosographic entity. The histochemical picture is often also characterized by type 1 fibre predominance, with hypotrophy of the same type of fibres in some cases (Gardner-Medwin, 1994).

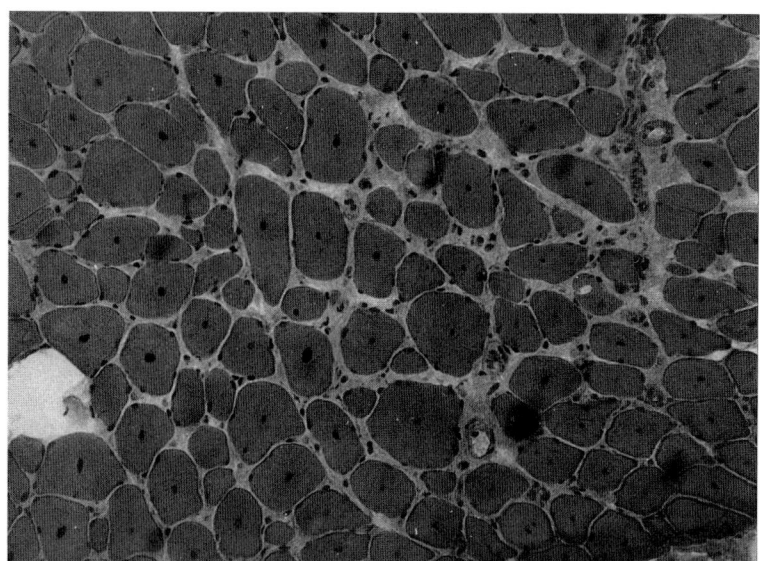

Fig. 1. Autosomal dominant myotubular/centronuclear myopathy: H & E (×200) stained frozen muscle sections show centrally located nuclei in almost all fibres.

From a clinical point of view, the usual form of this myopathy is characterized by varying degrees of muscular hypotonia and very slowly progressive weakness, evident in the neonatal period or later in childhood, often associated with external ophthalmoplegia. Some of the patients also present skeletal abnormalities such as foot deformities and scoliosis. As in our series of nine patients (Trevisan et al., 1986), serum CK is usually normal but EMG often shows myopathic features. Inheritance of this usual 'early infantile ophthalmoplegic form' of M/CM is generally considered to be autosomal recessive (Dubowitz, 1989; Wallgren-Pettersson, 1994). Since the study of McLeod et al. (1972) there has also been recognized a form of M/CM with a dominant mode of inheritance, and onset in adult life or childhood; in this form of M/CM external ophthalmoplegia is uncommon. A clear distinction, however, between the autosomal recessive and the dominant form of this congenital myopathy appears to be of dubious validity (Fardeau & Tomé, 1994; Gardner-Medwin, 1994): they could be different phenotypes of an autosomal dominant myopathy with reduced penetrance and variable clinical expression.

On both clinical and genetic grounds, however, the 'very severe X-linked' form is clearly distinguished from the autosomal type of the disease (Van Vijngardeen et al., 1969): in this variety of M/CM the males present a profound weakness in the perinatal period, with ventilatory insufficiency. Their mortality rate is more than 80 per cent in the first year of life (Bodensteiner, 1994). Genetic linkage analysis has localized the diaginic variant of M/CM to the proximal Xq28 region (Lehesjoki et al., 1990; Thomas et al., 1990).

In muscle, internal nuclei may be observed after denervation or in myotonic dystrophy. Differential diagnosis between congenital myotonic dystrophy and severe early onset M/CM may be difficult, requiring accurate neuromuscular evaluation of the neonate's mother.

The original controversial hypothesis of Spiro et al. (1966), that the muscular changes in M/CM could be an expression of an altered maturation of muscle fibres, has been found to be somehow valid in the X-linked type by immunocytochemical studies: Sawchack et al. (1991) found heavy chains of foetal myosin in muscle of this type of M/CM, and Sarnat (1992) detected an over-expression of vimentin and desmin intermediate filaments as in foetal myotubes. The same findings were not reported for the autosomal type of M/CM, apart from an over-expression of desmin (Figarella-Branger *et al.*, 1992; Mora *et al.*, 1994).

A few biochemical investigations have been carried out on M/CM. The identification of adenylate-cyclase deficiency in cultured muscle cells of two cases affected by the X-linked form of M/CM (Askanas *et al.*, 1979) seems in agreement with the immunocytochemical findings indicating the altered maturation of the muscle fibres.

Nemaline myopathy (NM)

This congenital myopathy was described in 1963 by Shy *et al.* and, independently, by Conen *et al.* The term 'nemaline' was used by Shy's group to indicate the thread-like bodies ('nema' is the Greek for thread) detected along the fibres. Electron microscopy evaluation of muscle biopsies of these patients subsequently showed a rod-like shape for the myogranules (Engel, 1966) and so NM was also named 'rod body myopathy'. Histochemically, the rods are evident by modified Gomori trichrome stain (see Fig. 2) as red-blueish irregular granulations. The rod bodies are mainly detected in type 1 fibres; moreover, a predominance of this type of fibre is considered characteristic of NM (Micaglio *et al.*, 1987; Middleton & Moser, 1994). Electron microscopy shows that the rod bodies are directly connected with the Z lines of the sarcomeres (Engel, 1966; Fardeau & Tomé, 1994), as lateral polymers mainly composed of alpha-actinin. The pathogenesis of these alterations of the Z line is not yet clarified, even if muscle deficiency of the enzyme dipeptidil-peptidase I, detected by Stauber *et al.* in two cases (1986), could play a role. This enzymatic deficit was not reported in other patients. Other biochemical data about NM were not useful to the understanding of its pathogenesis, such as the mild partial deficiency of free carnitine found in the serum of six of our patients (Trevisan *et al.*, 1986). Rod bodies in muscle, on the other hand, can be a secondary result of other pathology, such as tenotomy, denervation and inflammation, like that associated with HIV infection (Dwyer *et al.*, 1992; Goebel & Lenard, 1992; Gardner-Medwin, 1994). On clinical grounds, the manifestation of muscular involvement may be variable, even though the onset of NM

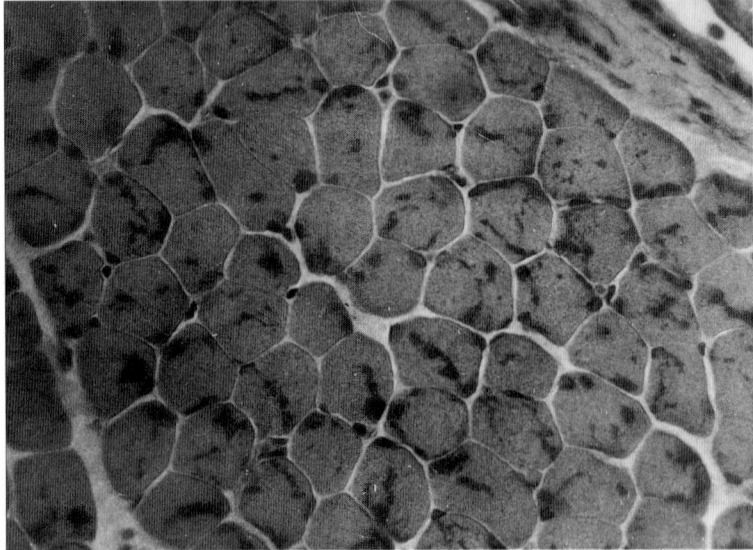

Fig. 2. Autosomal dominant nemaline myopathy: in the vast majority of muscle fibres, the trichrome stain (×200) gives evidence of the rods as irregular granular material.

is usually at birth with various degrees of muscular hypotonia and generalized weakness. In some cases there are severe ventilatory and swallowing difficulties. Two of our cases showed external ophthalmoplegia, but extraocular muscles are generally spared (Bodensteiner, 1994). Muscle involvement in this congenital myopathy is quite generalized with a slender appearance of the limbs; before the identification of the disease by the introduction of new adequate morphological techniques, some of these cases, such as the patient of Hopkins *et al.* (1966), were diagnosed as affected by 'Krabbe's universal muscle hypoplasia' (Ford, 1960). Some cases may show a progressive clinical course with death in childhood, such as in two of the seven patients studied by us (Trevisan *et al.*, 1986). More often, the muscle involvement in NM with early onset tends to be static or very slowly progressive. Patients with this myopathy often show a characteristic appearance with an elongated face, high arched palate, *pectus excavatum*, club-foot and kyphoscoliosis. Serum CK is usually normal, while an EMG, as in our patients, may show myopathic or also neuropathic features. In a sibling of one of our patients with neonatal onset of the disease, NM, ascertained by muscle biopsy, was asymptomatic, as was another case reported by Gonatas *et al.* in 1966: these patients with subclinical muscle involvement may eventually develop symptoms in adult life (Gardner-Medwin, 1994). Some authors (Meier *et al.*, 1984; Bodensteiner, 1994) distinguish the infantile type from the less frequent adult onset NM, in which cardiac involvement would be more frequent. However, the presence in the same family of patients with infantile onset of the symptoms and adults with subclinical expression, makes the separation of these two types of the disease questionable (Gardner-Medwin, 1994).

Autosomal dominant inheritance is generally recognized in this congenital myopathy, even if only in sporadic cases (Bodensteiner, 1994; Gardner-Medwin, 1994), and its gene has been shown to map to the q21–23 region of chromosome 1 (Laing *et al.*, 1992). The rare autosomal recessive form of NM appears linked to the 2q21–22 locus (Wallgren-Pettersson, 1995).

Central core disease (CCD)

As soon as histochemical techniques were used to evaluate muscle biopsies, this congenital myopathy was the first to be described, as originally reported by Shy & Magee (1956): in their patients trichrome staining showed in the vast majority of fibres around central areas of a blueish colour. A large number of cases were subsequently reported, with clear evidence that the pathognomonic features of the disease were central core images in cross-sections of type 1 fibres, devoid of oxidative enzymes (see Fig. 3). These oval formations, resulting from the lack of mitochondria, run through the length of the fibre: in the same areas myofibrillar architecture is often clearly altered. A common feature of CCD is also type 1 fibre predominance, as in nemaline and myotubular/centronuclear miopathies (Micaglio *et al.*, 1987; Middleton & Moser, 1994).

Pathogenesis of the cores in this congenital myopathy is unknown; however, core-like lesions may be determined by experimental tenotomy (Karpati *et al.*, 1972). A recent immunochemical investigation on cytoskeletal proteins of muscle from patients with CCD (Vita *et al.*, 1994), has shown over-expression of desmin intermediate filaments at the periphery of some cores, suggesting a possible role of this protein in core formation; the same alterations were not found in core-targetoid fibres due to denervation.

On clinical grounds, CCD is characterized by neonatal hypotonia, usually not severe, with a subsequent delay in motor milestones and evidence of permanent mild to moderate proximal weakness. Muscle involvement is usually static, even in instances of a slow progressive clinical course, as in one of five cases followed up by us (Trevisan *et al.*, 1986). Patients having CCD may present congenital hip dislocation or other skeletal abnormalities, as kyphoscoliosis. An onset in adult life with mild muscular weakness is very rare (Bodensteiner, 1994; Gardner-Medwin, 1994). In patients affected with CCD, serum CK and EMG are usually normal or mildly altered (Goebel

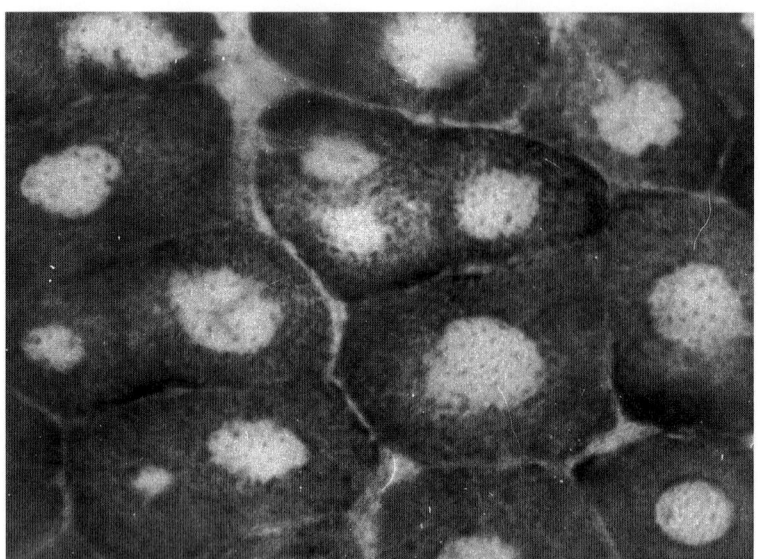

Fig. 3. Central core disease: in transverse section all the type 1 fibres have one or more central cores, the areas devoid of oxidative activity (NADH–TRP, ×330).

& Lenard, 1992; Fardeau & Tomé, 1994; Gardner-Medwin, 1994). Though some sporadic cases have been reported, CCD usually appears to be transmitted in an autosomal dominant mode, even if with a variable expression on both clinical and histopathological grounds; linkage genetic analysis by Haan *et al.* (1990) and Zhang *et al.* (1993) has mapped the gene of the disease to locus q13.1 of chromosome 19, with a possibility of being allelic to a gene for malignant hyperthermia. Susceptibility to this anaesthesiological risk has been recognized in patients affected by CCD for a long time.

Minicore or multicore disease

This is a congenital myopathy described in 1971 by Engel *et al.*, only apparently similar to CCD: actually the small and multifocal areas of degeneration characteristic of this disease may be found in both type 1 and type 2 muscle fibres and they usually run for only a few sarcomeres along them. They have a distinctive electron-microscopy, but their presence may also be aspecific and secondary to other myopathies (Bodensteiner, 1994). Usually, type 1 fibre predominance is also found in minicore disease.

The disease is generally evident in infancy, with mild and often non-progressive hypotonia and proximal weakness. Extraocular and facial muscles may be involved. Serum CK is normal and EMG is often of myopathic type. The mode of inheritance is mostly autosomal recessive (Dubowitz, 1989; Middleton & Moser, 1994) but autosomal dominant transmission is not excluded, at least in some families (Fardeau & Tomé, 1994).

Investigation of muscle biopsies of floppy infants in whom primary muscular or nervous disorders have not been detected, may show alterations in the normal histochemical mosaic of the muscle fibres. Type 1 fibre predominance (TIFP) is a not infrequent finding, but it may just be the incomplete pathological expression of the congenital myopathies that are well defined as NM, CCD and M/CM (Gardner-Medwin, 1994; Middleton & Moser, 1994; Wallgren-Pettersson, 1994). Follow up of 23 children with a diagnosis of TIFP (Kiriakides *et al.*, 1993) also showed that the change of muscle mosaic could be due to congenital muscular dystrophy, or to CNS or peripheral nerve pathology. The same study, however, showed that in 40 per cent of these patients TIFP appeared as a primary, even if aspecific, myopathy with a benign clinical course.

Another type of alteration of the muscle fibre mosaic is the so-called congenital fibre type disproportion (CFTD), a congenital myopathy described by Brooke in 1973 after re-evaluation of muscle biopsies from a series of children who suffered from infantile hypotonia of unknown origin. It is characterized by the average diameter of type 1 fibres being 12 per cent smaller than the normal one of type 2 fibres; type 1 fibres often predominate. In these patients, congenital hypotonia and weakness of various degrees are frequently associated with short stature, arthrogryposis, hip dislocation, high arched palate and other skeletal abnormalities. Serum CK may be slightly increased, EMG normal or mildly altered (Gardner-Medwin, 1994). The clinical evolution may be various, with a benign clinical course after the second year of life or with residual invaliding muscular weakness. The specific nosographic entity of this myopathy, however, is uncertain since the disproportion in fibre size may be a secondary finding for other neuromuscular disorders such as congenital myotonic dystrophy, infantile facioscapulo-humeral dystrophy, nemaline myopathy, or myotubular/centronuclear myopathy (Fardeau & Tomé, 1994). In a floppy infant diagnosed by muscle biopsy to be affected by CFTD, a subsequent postmortem re-evaluation of muscle pathology was suggestive of congenital muscular dystrophy (Cavanagh et al., 1979). With a stricter inclusion criterion – fibre 1 type diameter 50 per cent smaller than that of type 2 fibres – the nosographic entity of this congenital myopathy appears to be more consistent (Brooke, 1990). Its genetic transmission, according to Dubowitz (1989), is mainly autosomal recessive, but the autosomal dominant mode is also well proved (Bodensteiner, 1994).

Other forms of congenital myopathies with structural changes (Table 1) have been reported only occasionally and most of them are considered to be anecdotal findings of unclear meaning from a nosographic point of view. (Bodensteiner, 1994; Fardeau & Tomé, 1994).

Some of them, such as fingerprint body myopathy (Engel et al., 1972), may be identified only by electron microscopy, but others are also detected by routine histochemical stainings, such as reducing body myopathy (Brooke & Neville, 1972) or cap disease (Fidzianska et al., 1981).

Congenital myopathies of dystrophic type

Among congenital myopathies without structural changes, of major interest are congenital myotonic dystrophy and congenital muscular dystrophy. The latter form is a heterogeneous nosographic entity that the International Consortium on Congenital Muscular Dystrophy distinguishes as having four types: the classical form of Western countries, the Fukuyama type, the muscle–eye–brain disease and its variant, Walker–Warburg syndrome (Dubowitz, 1994). Their common presenting features are hypotonia and weakness of early onset, with variable dystrophic alterations in muscle. Recent immunocytochemical investigations (Tomé et al., 1994) have identified a subtype of the classical form with deficiency of laminin a-2 chain (merosin), a muscle protein of the extracellular matrix; the gene of this subtype of the disease has been localized to chromosome 6q22–23 by homozygosity mapping (Hillaire et al., 1994). The merosin-deficient subtype of classical congenital muscular dystrophy seems less frequent than the positive one: immunochemical evaluation of 18 of our patients with the classical form of the disease has shown complete deficiency of muscle merosin in four (Trevisan et al., 1995a, 1995b), partial deficiency in another, and normal amounts in the others. All the merosin-deficient cases had severe muscle involvement and subclinical white matter alterations at brain CT or magnetic resonance imaging (MRI), as originally found by Fardeau (1994). The muscular deficit was generally less severe in patients with normal muscle expression of merosin; moreover, some of these merosin-positive patients also presented minor brain abnormalities at neuroradiological evaluation (Trevisan et al., 1996).

The current nosography and the new ætiopathogenetic insights into congenital muscular dystrophy, arising from ongoing immunocytochemical and genetic investigations, are extensively discussed by Fardeau *et al.* in Chapter 3 of this book. The clinical, histochemical and genetic characteristics of congenital myotonic dystrophy are treated by Pizzuti *et al.* in Chapter 6.

Conclusions

Currently, congenital myopathies are generally considered to be genetic diseases with structural changes of muscle. However, myopathies of dystrophic or metabolic type with neonatal onset should also be classified in the same nosographic group. On clinical grounds, none of the congenital myopathies with structural changes shows pathognomic features, but some clinical characteristics may lead the clinician to the possible diagnosis of one of them, as the finding of skeletal abnormalities, such as high arched palate, foot and sternal deformities or hip dislocation is associated with hypotonia in a floppy infant. Hip dislocation seems to indicate particularly central core disease or congenital fibre type disproportion. Serum CK is usually normal in the congenital myopathies, whereas EMG, which is generally normal in central core disease, may often show alterations in nemaline myopathy and myotubular/centronuclear myopathy. The clinical course is considered benign, especially in central core disease. A severe and progressive muscle involvement, on the other hand, is characteristic of X-linked myotubular/centronuclear myopathy and it is also observed in some cases of nemaline myopathy. In any case, diagnosis of a specific congenital myopathy with structural changes may be defined only by evaluating the muscle biopsy with accurate histochemical stainings and electron microscopy.

The congenital myopathies often show a familial expression, with different possible modes of inheritance. Therefore an early specific diagnosis could allow correct genetic counselling of the child's family, other than correct clinical management of the patient.

Acknowledgements

Histological pictures shown in this chapter were kindly provided by Professor C. Angelini. Our work was supported by grants from Telethon-Italy (n. 688) and Italian CNR.

References

Askanas, V., Engel, W.K., Reddy, N.B. *et al.* (1979): X-linked recessive congenital muscle fiber hypotrophy with central nuclei. *Arch. Neurol.* **36**, 604–609.

Bodensteiner, J.B. (1994): Congenital myopathies. *Muscle Nerve* **17**, 131–144.

Brooke, M.H. (1973): Congenital fiber type disproportion. In: *Clinical studies in myology*, Part 2, ed. B.A. Kakulas, pp. 147–159. Amsterdam: Excerpta Medica.

Brooke, M.H. (1990): The congenital myopathies. *J. Neurol. Sci.* **98** (suppl), 401.

Brooke, M.H., Neville, H.E. (1972): Reducing body myopathy. *Neurology* **22**, 829–840.

Cavanagh, N.P.C., Lake, B.D. & McMenamin, P. (1979): Congenital fiber type disproportion myopathy: a histological diagnosis with an uncertain clinical outlook. *Arch. Dis. Child.* **54**, 735–743.

Conen, P.E., Murphy, E.G. & Donohue, W.L. (1963): Light and electron microscopic studies of 'myogranules' in a child with hypotonia and muscle weakness. *Can. Med. Assoc. J.* **89**, 983–986.

Dubowitz, V. (1989): A colour atlas of the muscle disorders in childhood. London: Wolfe.

Dubowitz, V. (1994): 22nd ENMC workshop report on congenital muscular dystrophy. *Neuromusc. Disord.* **4**, 75–81.

Dwyer, B.A, Mayer, R.F. & Lee, S.C. (1992): Progressive nemaline (rod) myopathy as a presentation of human immunodeficiency virus infection. *Arch. Neurol.* **49**, 440.

Engel, A.G. (1966): Late onset rod myopathy (a new syndrome?): light and electron microscopic observations in two cases. *Mayo Clin. Proc.* **41**, 713–741.

Engel, A.G., Angelini, C. & Gomez, M.R. (1972): Fingerprint body myopathy – a newly recognized congenital muscle disease. *Mayo Clin. Proc.* **47**, 377–388.

Engel, A.G., Gomez, M.R. & Groover, R.V. (1971): Multicore disease: a recently recognized congenital myopathy associated to multifocal degeneration of myopathy fibers. *Mayo Clin. Proc.* **46**, 666–681.

Fardeau, M. (1994): Clinical and immunocytochemical evidence of heterogeneity in classical congenital muscular dystrophy. In: *Proceedings of the International Symposium on Congenital Muscular Dystrophies*, ed. Y. Fukuyama, p. 5. Tokyo (Japan), July 8–9.

Fardeau, M. & Tomé, FM.S. (1994): Congenital myopathies. In: *Myology*, eds A.G. Engel & C. Franzini-Armstrong, pp. 1487–1532. New York: McGraw-Hill.

Fidzianska, A., Badurska, B., Ryniewicz, B. & Dembek, I. (1981): 'Cap disease': a new congenital myopathy. *Neurology* **31**, 1113–1120.

Figarella-Branger, D., Calore, E.E., Boucrault, J., Bianco, N., Rougon, G. & Pellissier, J.F. (1992): Expression of cell surface and cytoskeleton developmentally regulated proteins in adult centronuclear myopathies. *J. Neurol. Sci.* **109**, 69–76.

Ford, F.R. (1960): *Diseases of the nervous system in infancy, childhood and adolescence*. Springfield, IL: C.C. Thomas.

Gardner-Medwin, D. (1994): Neuromuscular disorders in infancy and childhood. In: *Disorders of voluntary muscles*, eds J. Walton, G. Karpati & D. Hilton-Jones, pp. 781–836. Edinburgh: Churchill Livingstone.

Goebel, H.H. & Lenard, H.G. (1992): Congenital myopathies. In: *Handbook of Clinical neurology, myopathies*, eds L.P. Rowland & S. Di Mauro, Vol. 18, pp. 331–367. Amsterdam: Elsevier.

Gonatas, N.K, Shy, G.M. & Godfrey, E.H. (1966): Nemaline myopathy: the origin of nemaline structures. *N. Engl. J. Med.* **274**, 535–539.

Haan, E.A., Freemantle, C.J., McCure, J.A., Friend, K.L. & Mulley, J.C. (1990): Assignment of the gene for central core disease to chromosome 19. *Hum. Genet.* **86**, 187–190.

Hillaire, D., Leclerc, A., Faure, S. *et al.* (1994): Localization of merosin-negative congenital muscular dystrophy of chromosome 6q2 by homozygosity mapping. *Hum. Mol. Genet.* **3**, 1657–1661.

Hopkins, I.J., Lindsey, J.R. & Ford, F.F. (1966): Nemaline myopathy. A long-term clinico-pathologic study of affected mother and daughter. *Brain* **89**, 299.

Karpati, G., Carpenter, S. & Eisen, A.A. (1972): Experimental core-like lesions and nemaline rods: a correlative morphological and physiological study. *Arch. Neurol.* **27**, 237–251.

Kiriakides, T., Silberstein, J.M., Jongpiputvanich, J. *et al.* (1993): The clinical significance of type 1 fiber predominance. *Muscle Nerve* **16**, 418–423.

Krabbe, K.H. (1958): Congenital generalized muscular atrophies. *Acta Psychiatr.* **33**, 94–99.

Laing, N.G., Majda, B.T., Akkari, P.A. *et al.* (1992): Assignment of a gene (NEMI) for autosomal dominant nemaline myopathy to chromosome 1. *Am. J. Hum. Genet.* **50**, 576–583.

Lehesjoki, A.E., Sankila, E.M., Miao, J. *et al.* (1990): X-linked neonatal myotubular myopathy: one recombination detected with four polymorphic DNA markers from Xq28. *J. Med. Genet.* **27**, 288–291.

McLeod, J.G., Baker, W. de C., Lethlean, A.K. & Shorey, C.P. (1972): Centronuclear myopathy with autosomal dominant inheritance. *J. Neurol. Sci.* **15**, 375–387.

Meier, C., Voellmy, W., Gertsch, M., Zimmermann, A. & Geissbuhler, J. (1984): Nemaline myopathy appearing in adults as cardiomyopathy: a clinicopathologic study. *Arch. Neurol.* **41**, 443–445.

Micaglio, G.F., Ceccato, M.B., Trevisan, C.P. & Angelini, C. (1987): Quantitative histopathology in congenital myopathies. *Riv. Neurol.* **57**, 261–263.

Middleton, L.T. & Moser, H. (1994): Rare neuromuscular disorders. In: *Diagnostic criteria for neuromuscular disorders*, ed. A.E.H. Emery, pp 70–72. Baarn (The Netherlands): ENMC.

Mora, M., Morandi, L., Merlini, L. *et al.* (1994): Fetus-like dystrophin expression and other cytoskeletal protein abnormalities in centronuclear myopathies. *Muscle Nerve* **17**, 1176–1184.

Mostacciuolo, M.L., Miorin, M., Martinello, F. *et al.* (1996): Genetic epidemiology of congenital muscular dystrophy in a sample from north-east Italy. *Hum. Genet.* **97**, 277–279.

Sarnat, H.B. (1992): Vimentin and desmin in maturing skeletal muscle and developmental myopathies. *Neurology* **42**, 1616–1624.

Sawchack, J.A., Sher, J.H., Norman, M.G., Kula, R.W. & Shafiq, S.A. (1991): Centronuclear myopathy heterogeneity: distinction of clinical types by myosin isoform patterns. *Neurology* **41,** 135–140.

Shy, G.M., Engel, W.K., Somers, J.E. & Wanko, T. (1963): Nemaline myopathy: a new congenital myopathy. *Brain* **86,** 793–810.

Shy, G.M. & Magee, K.R. (1956): A new congenital non-progressive myopathy. *Brain* 79, 610–621.

Spiro, A.J., Shy, G.M. & Gonatas, N.K. (1966): Myotubular myopathy: persistence of fetal muscle in an adolescent boy. *Arch. Neurol.* **14,** 1–14.

Stauber, W.T., Riggs, J.E., Schochet, S.S., Gutmann, L. & Crosby, T.W. (1986): Nemaline myopathy: evidence of dipeptidyl-peptidase I deficiency. *Arch. Neurol.* **43,** 39–41.

Thomas, N.S., Williams, H., Cole, G. *et al.* (1990): X-linked neonatal centronuclear/myotubular myopathy: evidence for linkage to Xq28 DNA marker loci. *J. Med. Genet.* **27,** 284–287.

Tomé, F.M.S, Evangelista, T. & Leclerc, A. (1994): Congenital muscular dystrophy with merosin deficiency. *C. R. Acad. Sci.* III **317,** 351–357.

Trevisan, C.P., Martinello, F., Fanin, M., *et al.* (1995a): Divergence of brain involvement in 22 cases with classical congenital muscular dystrophy: comparison between muscle merosin amount and neuroimaging data. *Ital. J. Neurol. Sci.* **16** (suppl.), 39.

Trevisan, C.P., Martinello, F., Ferruzza, E. & Angelini, C. (1995b): Divergence of central nervous system involvement in 2 Italian sisters with congenital muscular dystrophy: a clinical and neuroradiological follow-up. *Eur. Neurol.* **35,** 230–235.

Trevisan, C.P., Martinello, F., Ferruzza, E. *et al.* (1996): Brain alterations in the classical form of congenital muscular dystrophy: clinical and neuroimaging follow-up of 12 cases and correlation with expression of merosin in muscle. *Child. Nerv. Syst.* **12,** 604–610.

Trevisan, C.P., Micaglio, G.F., Segalla, P. & Angelini, C. (1986): Histomorphometric analysis, biochemical study and clinical follow-up in congenital myopathies. In: *X International Congress on Neuropathology, Stockholm,* p. 126.

Van Vijngardeen, G.K., Fleury, P., Bethlem, J. & Meijer, AEFH. (1969): Familial 'myotubular' myopathy. *Neurology* **19,** 901–908.

Vita, G., Migliorato, A. & Baradello, A. (1994): Expression of cytoskeleton proteins in central core disease. *J. Neurol. Sci.* **126,** 71–76.

Wallgren-Pettersson, C. (1994): Myotubular/centronuclear myopathy. In: *Diagnostic criteria for neuromuscular disorders,* ed. A.E.H. Emery, pp. 45–47. Baarn (The Netherlands): ENMC.

Wallgren-Pettersson, C., Avela, K., Marchand, S. *et al.* (1995): A gene for autosomal recessive nemalin myopathy assigned to chromosome 2q by linkage analysis. *Neuromusc. Disord,* **5,** 441–443.

Walton, J.N. (1956): Amyotonia congenita. A follow-up study. *Lancet* **i,** 1023.

Zhang, Y., Chen, H.S., Khanna, C.K. *et al.* (1993): A mutation in the human ryanodine receptor gene, associated with central core disease. *Nature Genetics* **5,** 46–51.

Chapter 6

The hereditary myotonic syndromes

Antonio Pizzuti,[1,2] Giuseppe Novelli[3] and Bruno Dallapiccola[2,3]

[1]*Institute of Neurology, University of Milan, Via F. Sforza 35, 20122 Milan, Italy;*
[2]*Ospedale C.S.S. San Giovanni Rotondo, Rome;*
[3]*Department of Public Health, Università Tor Vergata, 135 EdE Nord, 00133 Rome, Italy*

Summary

Myotonia, defined as difficulty in muscle relaxation after effort, is a symptom common to many different diseases. Many myotonic syndromes have a hereditary origin. Myotonia as a symptom seems to derive from derangements of the muscle membrane ion distribution. Hereditary myotonias may be divided in two groups, dystrophic and non-dystrophic forms. While the first actually comprises only one disease (myotonic dystrophy, by far the most common form of myotonia), the second (non-dystrophic) may be further divided into two sub-groups, i.e. the chloride channel disease group (mutations in a chloride ion channel gene) and the sodium channel group (mutations in a sodium ion channel gene). The chloride channel disorders comprise paramyotonia congenita, myotonia fluctuans and hyperkalaemic periodic paralysis. The chloride channel disorders comprise both the autosomal and the recessive forms of congenital myotonia.

The myotonic dystrophy (DM) gene does not code for an ion channel, but for a protein-kinase, whose function is still unknown. DM exhibits a peculiar mutation mechanism. An unstable CTG triplet repeat, present at the 3′ non-coding region of the mRNA, expands in DM patients. The length of the expanded repeat has a direct relationship to the severity of the disease. The mutation mechanism helps explain such phenomena as clinical anticipation, expression variability and the exclusive transmission of the severe congenital form through affected mothers.

Myotonia (MY) may be defined as a delayed muscle relaxation after both voluntary contraction and mechanical or electrical stimulation. MY is recorded by electromyography as a repetitive high-frequency discharge (20–80 Hz) of single fibre potentials due to a sustained electrical activity at the muscle membrane (Landau, 1952). Indeed, the clinical phenomenon arises from abnormalities in the muscle membranes, bringing about changes in the distribution and movement of electrical charges across the membrane itself (Lanari, 1946).

MY patients complain of stiffness in their muscles during the myotonic contraction, usually without pain. Most patients report some relief of the stiffness after exercise (warm-up phenomenon). However, in rare cases, MY may also increase during muscle activity (paradoxical MY).

MY must be distinguished by other similar but unrelated clinical phenomena not originating in the muscle membrane. First, MY is not abolished by blockage of the neuromuscular junction, as in neuromyotonic discharge (Isaacs' syndrome) (Isaacs, 1961) and myokymia (Satoyoshi, 1972), both originating from motor nerves and their terminal endings. MY is also unaffected by drugs which decrease the synaptic transmission in the spinal cord (e.g. benzodiazepines). MY must also be distinguished from silent contractures, a typical symptom of some metabolic disorders (Di Mauro et al., 1984).

MY is not a disease. It is a symptom, common to several hereditary and acquired conditions (Table 1). This review will focus on those hereditary syndromes, where the genetic mutation mechanism has been elucidated, contributing new insights to the pathophysiology of MY. However, a few words on other MYs are necessary. Beside genetic causes, drugs and toxins are the most likely agents causing MY. A myotonic syndrome may be caused in normal individuals by the herbicide 2,4-dichlorophenoxyacetate (2,4-D) (Pohl, 1917). This compound specifically blocks chloride conductance (Palade & Barchi, 1977). Myotonia has also been observed after the treatment of hypercholesterolaemia with 20,25-diazacholesterol (20,25-D) (Winer et al., 1966). This drug inhibits the conversion of demosterol to cholesterol. It has been observed that the resulting changes in viscosity of muscle membranes also reduces the chloride conductance (Chalikian & Barchi, 1980).

In general the genetic disorders with MY may be divided in two groups: dystrophic MY (myotonic dystrophy (DM) and chondrodystrophic MY (CDMY)) and the non-dystrophic MY (Table 1).

Table 1. Disorders associated with myotonia

Hereditary disorders
(a) Dystrophic myotonias
  Myotonic dystrophy (Steinert) AD
  Chondrodystrophic myotonia (Schwartz–Jampel) AR (rare AD)
(b) Non-dystrophic myotonias
  (1) Chloride channel disorders
    Paramyotonia congenita (Eulemburg) AD
    Hyperkalaemic paralysis periodica (Garmstorp) AD
    Myotonia fluctuans AD
  (2) Sodium channel disorders
    Dominant myotonia congenita (Thomsen) AD
    Recessive generalized myotonia (Becker) AR

Acquired disorders
  Aromatic carboxylic acids
  Cholesterol synthesis inhibitors

Non-dystrophic myotonias

Based on the molecular mutation mechanisms, the non-dystrophic myotonias may be further divided in two groups: chloride channel and sodium channel diseases. As a group, these disorders are quite rare. Their study is important, however, in collecting information on the molecular and physiological features of myotonia, aiming at a more specific rationale for symptomatic drug treatment.

To understand the mechanisms through which derangement in ion channel function can affect muscle membrane excitability, the membrane's electrical proprieties must be reviewed.

The muscle membrane resting potential is determined by two main factors: the distribution of the ion charges across the membrane, which is the result of active transport, and their relative membrane permeability (conductance) through specific ion channels. At rest, the muscle membrane is largely permeable to chloride ions (Cl^-) and, at a lesser extent, to potassium (K^+). The membrane is almost impermeable to sodium (Na^+). The relative ion conductance explains why the membrane resting potential is shifted toward the equilibrium potential of Cl^- and K^+. When a depolarizing stimulus reaches a threshold, it is sensed by the Na⁺ channels, which open, allowing Na⁺ to flow into the cell. The increase of Na⁺ conductance shifts the membrane potential toward the potential equilibrium for Na⁺ (positive inside), further depolarizing the membrane. After that, the Na⁺ channels close and the K⁺ channels open, causing the membrane to repolarize.

Abnormalities in Na⁺ channels can lead to repetitive action potential discharges as seen in MY. After the membrane repolarizes, following an action potential, for some time normal Na⁺ channels cannot open again (refractory period). An increase in the rate of recovery can reduce the refractory period and open the Na⁺ channels before the membrane is fully repolarized, resulting in bursts of action potentials.

The sodium channel myotonias

Paramyotonia congenita (PC) (Eulemberg, 1986; Becker, 1977)

PC is an autosomal dominant disorder. Patients complain of MY, which is greatly increased by cold. In some cases, there is no MY in warm environments. Exposure to cold first produces MY and, if unrelieved, muscle weakness very similar to the flaccid paralysis of periodic paralysis patients. Rewarming can stop both MY and paralysis. The disorder does not progress. Facial MY is quite typical. PC shows paradoxical MY, and paralytic episodes can be induced by exercise. As detailed later on, PC is clinically very similar to hyperkalaemic periodic paralysis (hyper-PP) and indeed PC and hyper-PP are allelic mutations.

Hyperkalaemic periodic paralysis (hyper-PP) (Gamstorp, 1963)

The periodic paralyses are characterized by attacks of weakness associated with loss of muscle membrane excitability. Paralytic episodes are often heralded by changes in the serum K⁺ concentration, which may decrease (hypokalaemic-PP), increase (hyperkalaemic-PP) or remain normal (normokalaemic-PP). Hyper-PP can be associated with myotonic features. The disorder is autosomal dominant. In some families MY is not present, while in others it is only triggered by cold, resembling PC. Hyper-PP syndromes and PC are due to mutations in the same sodium channel gene.

Myotonia fluctuans (MF) (Ricker et al., 1990)

MF is a rare autosomal dominant form of myotonia, characterized by wide temporal variation of MY. Typically, MY is often accompanied by pain. MF is not progressive and in some respects resembles the chloride channel MYs. However, mutation in the same gene as PC and HyperPP have been reported.

Hyper-PP and PC genes have been mapped to chromosome 17, close to the growth hormone gene (Ebers et al., 1990). A sodium ion channel alpha-subunit gene was mapped in the same region (SCN4A) (Fontaine et al., 1990), very similar to a cat homology. Hyper-PPs, PC and MF are due to different mutations at this locus (Ptacek et al., 1991, 1992). SCN4A is a specifically expressed gene for skeletal muscle, spanning 30 Kb in the chromosome 17q23 region (Ptacek et al., 1992). Ten other ion channel alpha-subunit genes have been isolated so far, with different tissue specificities. Depending on the specific mutation, SCN4A extreme and intermediate phenotypes are generated. Most mutations are concentrated in exons 22–24, corresponding to the activation sites of the channel (McClatchey et al., 1992). At present, it is not possible to predict if a specific mutation will always lead to periodic weakness, muscle stiffness, muscle paralysis after exposure to cold, or sensitivity to potassium loading.

The chloride channel myotonias

Abnormalities in chloride ion conductance can also generate MY. As mentioned above, a reduction in chloride conductance is the mechanism through which both 2,4-D and 20,25-D can cause MY. Low Cl⁻ conductance is also the defect in the myotonic *adr* mouse mutant (Rudel, 1990). MY develops when the Cl⁻ conductance is reduced more than 80 per cent (Barchi, 1975). As mentioned above, Cl⁻ conductance represents most of the muscle resting membrane conductance. During the action potential small amounts of Na^+ and K^+ move across the membrane. Within the muscle fibre, ion movement does not appreciably change the cytoplasmic ion concentration, due to the large intracellular volume compared to the number of moving molecules. Into the narrow T-tubular system, however, the released K^+ can raise its intraluminal concentration up to 0.3 mM after a single action potential. In normal muscle, the depolarizing effect of intraluminal K^+ increase is shunted by the large Cl⁻ conductance. If Cl⁻ conductance is severely decreased, K^+ accumulation can actually depolarize the T-tubule, causing sequential action potential discharges. Reduction of the Cl⁻ conductance due to Cl⁻ channel mutation is the pathophysiological mechanism common to the chloride channel myotonias.

Dominant congenital myotonia (DCM) (Thomsen, 1876)

DCM is the dominant form of chloride channel myotonic syndromes. MY is generalized, but symptoms are not progressive, differing from the recessive form. MY is often present at birth. Symptoms are more frequent in lower limbs, followed by hands and facial muscles. Disease onset is always earlier than 6 years. MY does not fluctuate and is not affected by cold. Continued exercise can reduce stiffness (warm-up phenomenon). Muscular hypertrophy is common in these patients (athletic habitus).

Recessive generalized myotonia (RGM) (Becker, 1973)

The onset is a little later than DMC (between 6 and 12 years old), with a similar muscle distribution. Differing from DMC, RGM patients may complain of an increasing severity of symptoms through the years. Almost 50 per cent of RGM patients show muscle weakness, which can also increase in severity. Muscular hypertrophy is more common and dramatic in RGM than in DMC (Herculean habitus). In the past, RGM was often considered as an intermediate phenotype between DMC and DM. It is now clear that RGM and DMC are allelic hereditary disorders. It is worth noting that different mutations in the same gene may have either dominant or recessive effects on the resulting phenotype.

DMC and RGM genes have both been mapped by linkage analysis at the same chromosome 7 locus, close to the T-cell beta receptor. The mutated gene is a skeletal muscle chloride channel gene (CHLCN1) (Koch *et al.*, 1992, George *et al.*, 1993). The mouse homologous gene is mutated in the myotonic *adr* mouse. CHCL1 is a member of a larger chloride channel gene family responsible for most (80 per cent) of the chloride conductance in skeletal muscles.

A few words must be added on a calcium channel disorder (hypokalaemic paralysis periodica), where episodic weakness is not associated to MY.

The calcium channel disorders

Hypokalaemic periodic paralysis (Hypo-PP)

Hypo-PP is an autosomal dominant disorder with onset after the second decade of life. Patients present with acute and reversible attacks of muscle weakness accompanied by a fall in blood of potassium levels. Muscle weakness during attacks is due to the persistent depolarization of the sarcolemmal membrane. The hypo-PP locus maps to chromosome 1q31–32 within the interval also containing the DHP-sensitive calcium channel alpha-1 subunit. Mutations in this gene were recently found in patients with hypo-PP. However, linkage analysis has also revealed unlinked families, suggesting genetic heterogeneity for this disease.

Dystrophic myotonic syndromes

This disease group is virtually made up of patients with the most common form of myotonic syndrome, i.e. DM. Another, far rarer hereditary disease, chondrodystrophic myotonia (CDMY) (Schwartz & Jampel, 1962) will be briefly described.

CDMY is characterized by dwarfism, skeletal abnormalities, MY and characteristic facial features. It is an autosomal recessive disorder (some dominant families have also been reported), without progression. The disorder appears within the first year. Twenty per cent of patients show mental retardation. Skeletal dysmorphisms are the dystrophyc changes which the disease name refers to.

Myotonic dystrophy

DM is an autosomal dominant disease. It is the most common muscular dystrophy (1:8000 prevalence). As its name indicates, the main features of DM are muscle atrophy and MY. However, DM may be considered a multi-systemic disease also affecting the heart (conduction defects), the endocrine glands (male hypogonadism), the skin (precocious baldness), the eye (cataracts) and many other organs (Harper, 1989). Genetically, DM is characterized by variable expression, since its severity varies from very mild late-onset cases, with precocious baldness, cataracts and light muscle involvement to the most severe congenital form (CDM), characterized by neonatal floppiness, muscle involvement and mental retardation (Harper, 1989). Interestingly, CDM is almost always transmitted by affected mothers, and exceptionally by fathers. Effects on single organs may also vary among patients, even in the same family (Harper, 1989).

The gene responsible for DM has been assigned, by linkage analysis, to the long arm of chromosome 19, and then isolated by positional cloning (Ashizawa & Hejtmanncik, 1990). The gene codes for a serine/threonine protein kinase, whose function is still unknown. The DM gene exhibits a peculiar mutation mechanism. It contains an unstable triplet repeat that can mitotically and/or meiotically change its length (expansion), disrupting the kinetics of gene transcription and the level of the resulting protein (Fu et al., 1993).

This mutation mechanism is common to other neurological disorders including the fragile X syndrome (FRAXA) (Verkerk et al., 1991), the mental retardation syndrome with fragile X type E (FRAXE) (Knight et al., 1993), Kennedy's disease (SBMA) (La Spada et al., 1991), Huntington disease (HD) (HD collaborative group, 1993), spinocerebellar ataxia type 1 (SCA1) (Orr et al., 1993), dentatorubro-pallidoluysian atrophy or Haw River syndrome (DRPLA) (Koide et al., 1994) and Machado–Joseph disease (MJD). As a group they are now referred as the triplet repeat diseases (Caskey et al., 1992).

As mentioned above, DM patients show large variability in disease severity. The phenotype is related to quantitative features of the mutation. Larger expansions result in more severe phenotypes. The larger the triplet repeat in the mutated alleles, the more severe the disease. It is clear that DM diagnosis can be obtained by measuring the triplet repeat in the DM gene, by PCR or Southern blotting.

Molecular biology of the DM gene

The DM gene transcribes a 3.2 kb mRNA from 15 exons distributed over 13 kb of genomic DNA (Fu et al., 1993). The gene product, a 624 amino acid protein, is highly homologous to cAMP-dependent protein kinases, and it has been therefore called myotonin-protein kinase (MT-PK) (Brook et al., 1992; Fu et al., 1993). Little is actually known on MT-PK function and subcellular distribution. MT-PK is able to phosphorylate both tyrosine residues in skeletal muscle and the beta subunit of the DHPD receptor. Preliminary evidence suggests that MT-PK may be either involved in regulating synaptic signal transmission or in assembling the neuromuscular junctions (Wieringa, 1994). MT-PK mRNA has been recovered from different tissues, in humans and in mice (Brook et al., 1992). It is mostly concentrated in the heart (in particular the conduction system), the skeletal muscle and the central nervous system. Several spliced mRNA forms have been identified both in humans and mice (Fu et al., 1993; Jansen et al., 1994). However, a single peptide of 53 kDa in skeletal muscle and brain, and a 62 kDa protein in cardiac muscle (Brewster et al., 1993; Fu et al., 1993) have been detected by Western blotting.

The mutation mechanism

The 3' exon of the MT-PK gene contains a polymorphic CTG triplet repeat (Brook et al., 1992; Fu et al., 1992). Normal individuals show alleles with a variable CTG triplet repeat number (usually from five to less than 50 elements) (Brunner et al., 1992). The alleles containing more than 50 CTGs are considered to be mutated and cause DM (Fu et al., 1992). General population analysis demonstrated high heterozygosity of the repeat length (0.75–0.80), with a non-random allele distribution (Brook et al., 1992; Fu et al., 1992; Davies et al., 1992). The five-repeat allele, for instance, shows 8–22 per cent frequency, while alleles with more than 19 repeats are found only in about 5 per cent of Caucasian and Japanese populations (Davies et al., 1992).

Repeats in the normal range appear to be quite stable. By contrast, expanded triplet repeats are unstable. Their tendency to further expand increases with their length. Unstable repeats change the length during DNA replication processes, before mitosis and meiosis.

Population studies indicate that all the DM expanded alleles derive from a very small number of original mutations, possibly only one (Imbert et al., 1993; Neville et al., 1994). The founder event(s) consisted in a jump from an allele with five repeats to one with 19–30 repeats. Alleles with 19–30 repeats may still be the reservoir for recurrent DM mutations. In fact, sub-Saharan people, in whom DM is apparently rare, lack these 'normal' alleles (Novelli et al., 1994).

In other disorders, but not in DM, factors intrinsic to the gene, other than the repeat length, can affect the stability of the repeat itself. They include breaks in pure triplet repeats, as observed in SCA1 and FRAXA (Banfi et al., 1994). The transition from stable and/or ancestral short alleles to the 'critical' 19–37 range alleles in DM involved some mechanism(s) different than those of other triplet repeat diseases. Meiotic drive is evident at the DM locus, favouring the transmission of the predisposing and disease-causing alleles (Gennarelli et al., 1995).

Clinical–genetic relationships

Genetic anticipation is present when the clinical severity of a hereditary disease increases through generations of the same family (Harper, 1989). For a long time, anticipation was considered by geneticists to be the result of ascertainment bias (Penrose, 1948). In DM, however, there is no doubt of its occurrence, and its relation to the mode of transmission for the mutated alleles. Within families showing anticipation, the triplet repeat generally increases its length, as may be demonstrated by Southern blotting analysis of genomic DNA. Anticipation by progressive allele expansion is a consistent feature in DM families, observed in more than 90 per cent of cases (Ashizawa et al., 1992; Redman, 1993).

The relentless process of progressive expansion of the unstable repeat occurs asynchronously in different affected branches of the same family. This phenomenon would eventually lead to the complete loss of the mutated allele. The high frequency of the mutated allele can be accounted for only by the presence of a pool of asymptomatic families carrying 'at risk' alleles.

Another source of new DM alleles are the contracted repeats in fully expressing families (Ashizawa et al., 1994; Brunner et al., 1993; Redman et al., 1993). Contraction of the CTG repeat towards the normal range occurs in about 6 per cent of parent–child pairs studied. It preferentially occurs in male transmission (Ashizawa et al., 1993). As is expected in some contracting parent–child pairs, the disease severity decreases in the second generation. However, anticipation is still present in 48 per cent of these pairs. It is evident that the DNA expansion is not the sole determinant of the clinical outcome.

Why do repeat contractions preferentially occur in alleles transmitted by fathers? Lavedan et al. (1993) described a series of 91 father–child pairs. Paternal repeats expanded only when the repeat was less than 2 kb. Repeats longer than 1.5 kb contracted. Male gametes seem unable to keep triplet repeats whose length is associated with the transmission of CDM, explaining why CDM is only transmitted by affected mothers.

Genotype–phenotype correlation studies have largely pointed at the age of onset of the disease, and have demonstrated that the increase of the triplet repeat length positively correlates to the clinical severity (Tsilfidis et al., 1992). The same relation pertains to most of the single symptom, typical of DM. The best correlation with the triplet repeat has been found in muscle weakness. Among the other clinical manifestations (Novelli et al., 1994b), heart findings (Melancini et al., 1994) (complete left bundle branch block and ventricular late potential), and endocrinological signs (levels of LH and FSH and male hypogonadism) revealed a significant correlation with the CTG repeat size. The correlation with ocular symptoms (unilateral and bilateral cataracts –Novelli et al., 1993a) is less clear. Even for other parameters (e.g. IQ) the correlation does not seem so tight.

In general, the correlation between genotype and phenotype holds for most patients. However, new data indicate that the triplet repeat status is not the only determinant of the symptom severity in DM. Genetic modifiers may be at work. DM families have been described, where similar CTG expansion ranges in different patients cause different clinical manifestations (Novelli et al., 1993b).

Many similar case reports demonstrate that the repeat size cannot always be a reliable predictor of the phenotype. First of all, the repeat length range in late onset, juvenile/adult and congenital forms of the disease is wide and overlapping. Second, discrepancies in genotype–phenotype correlation may be found in families with triplet repeat regression, where the child with contracted repeats still 'anticipates' the disease onset.

In many cases, those discrepancies are only apparent and due to somatic mosaicism in the CTG length. The expanded triplet repeat in DM patients is so unstable during mitotic events as to bring many tissues to a high degree of somatic mosaicism. Mosaicism is better observed in genomic Southern blotting where a hybridization smear corresponding to many triplet repeat lengths in leukocytes is common. The same smeary appearance is also observed when other tissue DNAs are analysed. The triplet repeat range may also differ in different tissues of the same patient (Ashizawa et al., 1993; Massari et al., 1995; Thornton et al., 1994).

Differences in single organ affects probably depend on differences in tissue-specific expansion ranges. Furthermore, different tissues show a different tendency toward expansion. Skeletal muscle expands 2–13 times more than leukocytes (Thornton et al., 1994) and the heart more than fibroblasts or liver (Jansen et al., 1994). As reported above, sperm cells cannot expand over 1000–1500 CTG triplets (Jansen et al., 1994).

Muscles derived from different myotomes show the same expansion range (Massari et al., 1995; Thornton et al., 1994) as different regions of the encephalon (frontal cortex and thalamus). Thus, the origin of this somatic mosaicism is probably at early embryonic stages. Afterwards, the mutated repeat seems to be stable as demonstrated by studies on identical twins.

It is anyway clear that other factors are responsible for the phenotypic expression of the disease and that the prognostic value of the direct DNA diagnosis of DM must be very critically considered.

References

Ashizawa, T. & Hejtmanncik, J.F. (1990): Myotonic dystrophy. *Curr. Neurol.* **10**, 27–62.

Ashizawa, T. *et al.* (1992): Anticipation in myotonic dystrophy: complex relationships between clinical findings and structure of the CGT repeat. *Neurology* **4**, 1877–1883.

Ashizawa, T. *et al.* (1993): Somatic instability of CTG repeat in myotonic dystrophy. *Neurology* **43**, 2674–2678.

Ashizawa, T. *et al.* (1994): Characteristics of intergenerational contractions of the CTG repeat in myotonic dystrophy. *Am. J. Hum. Genet.* **54**, 414–423.

Banfi, S. *et al.* (1994): Identification and characterization of the gene causing type 1 spinocerebellar ataxia. *Nature Genet.* **7**, 513–519.

Barchi, R.L. (1975): Myotonia: an evaluation of the chloride hypotesis. *Arch. Neurol.* **32**, 175–180.

Becker, P.E. (1973): Generalized non-dystrophic myotonia. The dominant (Thomsen) type and the recently identified recessive type. In: *New developments in electromyography and clinical neurophysiology*, eds J.E. Desmedt, pp. 407–412. Basel: Karger.

Becker, P.E. (1977): *Myotonia congenita and syndromes associated with myotonia*. Stuttgart: Thieme.

Brewster, B.S. *et al.* (1993): Identification of a protein product of the myotonic dystrophy gene using peptide specific antibodies. *Biochem. Biophys. Res. Commun.* **194**, 1256–1360.

Brook, J.D. *et al.* (1992): Molecular basis of myotonic dystrophy: expansion of a trinucleotide (CTG) repeat at the 3' end of a transcript encoding a protein kinase family member. *Cell* **68**, 799–808.

Brunner, H.G. *et al.* (1992): Presymptomatic diagnosis of myotonic dystrophy. *J. Med. Genet.* **29**, 780–784.

Brunner, H.G. *et al.* (1993): Reverse mutation in myotonic dystrophy. *N. Engl. J. Med.* **238**, 476–480.

Caskey, C.T. *et al.* (1992): Triplet repeat mutation in human disease. *Science* **256**, 784–789.

Chalikian, D.M. & Barchi, R.L. (1980): 20,25-diazacholesterol myotonia: biochemical characteristics of the sarcolemma. *Neurology* **30**, 423–424.

Davies, J. *et al.* (1992): Comparison of the myotonic dystrophy associated CTG repeat in European and Japanese populations. *J. Med. Genet.* **29**, 766–769.

Di Mauro, S. *et al.* (1984): Disorders of glycogen metabolism in muscle. *CRC Crit. Rev. Clin. Neurobiol.* **1**, 83–116.

Ebers, B. *et al.* (1990): Paramyotonia congenita and hyperkalemic periodic paralysis are linked to the adult muscle sodium channel gene. *Ann. Neurol.* **30**, 810–816.

Eulemberg, A. (1986): Über eine familiäre, durch 6 Generationen verfolgbare Form congenitaler Paramyotonie. *Neurol. Zentralbl.* **12**, 265–272.

Fontaine, B. *et al.* (1990): Hyperkalemic periodic paralysis and the adult muscle sodium channel alpha-subunit gene. *Science* **250**, 1000–1002.

Fu, Y.-H. *et al.* (1992): An unstable triplet repeat in a gene related to the myotonic dystrophy. *Science* **55**, 1256–1258.

Fu, Y.-H. *et al.* (1993): Varying expression of myotonin protein kinase mRNA and protein levels in the adult form of myotonic dystrophy. *Science* **72**, 971–983.

Gamstorp, I. (1963): Adynamia episodica hereditaria. *Acta Neurol. Scand.* **39**, 41–58.

Gennarelli, M. *et al.* (1995): Meiotic drive at the myotonic dystrophy locus. *J. Med. Genet.* **31**, 980.

George, A.L. *et al.* (1993): Molecular basis of Thomsen disease (autosomal dominant myotonia congenita). *Nature Genet.* **3**, 305–310.

Harper, P.S. (1989): *Myotonic dystrophy*. Philadelphia: W.B. Saunders.

Huntington's Disease Collaborative Research Group (1993): A novel gene containing a trinucleotide repeat that is expanded and unstable in Huntington's disease chromosomes. *Cell* **72**, 971–983.

Imbert, G. *et al.* (1993): Origin of the expansion-mutation in myotonic dystrophy. *Nature Genet.* **4**, 72–76.

Isaacs, H. (1961): A syndrome of continuous muscle-fiber activity. *J. Neurol. Neurosurg. Psychiatry* **24**, 319–325.

Jansen, G. *et al.* (1994): Gonosomal mosaicism in myotonic dystrophy patients: involvement of mitotic event in (CTG)n repeat variation and selection against extreme expansion on sperm. *Am. J. Hum. Genet.* **54**, 575–585.

Knight, S.J.L. *et al.* (1993): Trinucleotide repeat amplification and hypermethylation of a CpG island in FRAXE mental retardation. *Cell* **74**, 127–134.

Koch, M.C. et al. (1992): The skeletal muscle chloride channel in dominant and recessive human myotonia. *Science* **257**, 797–800.

Koide, R. et al. (1994): Unstable expansion of CAG repeat in hereditary dentatorubral-pallidoluysian atrophy (DPRLA). *Nature Genet.* **6**, 9–13.

La Spada, A. et al. (1991): Androgen receptor gene mutation in X-linked spinal and bulbar muscular atrophy. *Nature* **352**, 77–79.

Lanari, A. (1946): Mechanism of myotonic contraction. *Science* **104**, 221–222.

Landau, W.M. (1952): The essential mechanism in myotonia: an electromyographic study. *Neurology* **2**, 369–388.

Lavedan, C. et al. (1993): Different sex-dependent constraints in CTG length variation as explanation for congenital myotonic dystrophy. *Lancet* **341**, 237.

Massari, A. et al. (1995): Postzygotic instability of the myotonic dystrophy p(AGC)n repeat supported by larger expansions in muscle and reduced amplifications in sperm. *J. Neurol.* **242**, 379–383.

McClatchey, A. et al. (1992): Temperature-sensitive mutations in the II–IV cytoplasmatic loop region of the skeletal muscle sodium channel gene in paramyotonia congenita. *Cell* **68**, 769–774.

Melancini, P. et al. (1994): Correlation between cardiac involvement and CTG trinucleotide repeat length in myotonic dystrophy. *J. Am. Coll. Cardiol.* **25**, 239–245.

Neville, C. et al. (1994): High resolution genetic analysis suggests one ancestral predisposing haplotype for the origin of the myotonic dystrophy mutation. *Hum. Mol. Genet.* **1**, 45–51.

Novelli, G. et al. (1993a): Failure in detecting mRNA transcripts from the mutated allele in myotonic dystrophy muscle. *Biochem. Mol. Biol. Int.* **29**, 291–297.

Novelli, G. et al. (1993b): (CTG)n triplet mutation and phenotype manifestations in myotonic dystrophy patients. *Biochem. Med. Met. Biol.* **50**, 85–92.

Novelli, G. et al. (1994a): High conservation of the trinucleotide (CTG)n repeat at the myotonic dystrophy locus in nonhuman primates. *Hum. Evol.* **4**, 315–321.

Novelli, G. et al. (1994b): North Eurasian origin of the myotonic dystrophy mutation. *Hum. Mutat.* **4**, 79–81.

Orr, H.T. et al. (1993): Expansion of an unstable trinucleotide CAG repeat in spinocerebellar ataxia type 1. *Nature Genet.* **4**, 221–226.

Palade, P.T. & Barchi, R.L. (1977): On the inhibition of muscle membrane chloride conductances by aromatic carboxylic acids. *J. Gen. Physiol.* **69**, 875–896.

Penrose, L.S. (1948): The problem of anticipation in pedigrees of dystrophia myotonica. *Ann. Eugen.* **14**, 125–232.

Pizzuti, A. et al. (1993): The myotonic dystrophy gene. *Arch. Neurol.* **50**, 173–1179.

Pohl, J. (1917): Physiologische Wirkung des Hydroatophans. *Z. Exp. Pathol. Ther.* **19**, 198–204.

Ptacek, L.J. et al. (1991): Identification of a mutation in a gene causing hyperkalemic periodic paralysis. *Cell* **67**, 159–165.

Ptacek, L.J. et al. (1992): Mutation in a S4 segment of the adult skeletal muscle sodium channel cause paramyotonia congenita. *Neuron* **8**, 891–897.

Redman, J. et al. (1993): Relationship between parental trinucleotide GCT repeat length and clinical severity in offsprings. *JAMA* **269**, 1960–1965.

Ricker, K.F. et al. (1990): Myotonia fluctuans. *Arch. Neurol.* **47**, 268–272.

Rudel, R. (1990): The myotonic mouse: a realistic model of human recessive generalized myotonia. *Trend Neurosci.* **1**, 1–3.

Satoyoshi, E.Y. et al. (1972): Pseudomyotonia in cervical root lesions with myelopathy. A sign of the misdirection of regenerating nerve. *Arch. Neurol.* **27**, 307–313.

Schwartz, O. & Jampel, R.S. (1962): Congenital blepharophimosis associated with a unique generalized myopathy. *Arch. Ophthalmol.* **68**, 52–57.

Thomsen, J. (1876): Tonische Krampfe in willkürlich beweglichen Muskeln in Folge von ererbter psychischer Disposition. *Arch. Psychiatr.* **6**, 702–718.

Thornton, C.A. et al. (1994): Myotonic dystrophy patients have larger expansions in skeletal muscle than in leukocytes. *Ann. Neurol.* **35**, 104–107.

Tsilfidis, C. (1992): Correlation between CTG trinucleotide repeat length and frequency of severe congenital myotonic dystrophy. *Nature Genet.* **1,** 192–195.

Verkerk, A.J.M.H. *et al.* (1991): Identification of a gene (FMR-1) containing a CGG repeat coincident with a break-point cluster region exhibiting length variation in fragile-X syndrome. *Cell* **65,** 905–914.

Wieringa, B. (1994): Myotonic dystrophy reviewed: back to the future? *Hum. Mol. Genet.* **3,** 1–7.

Winer, N. *et al.* (1966): Myotonic response induced by inhibitors of cholesterol biosynthesis. *Science* **153,** 312–313.

Chapter 7

Hereditary motor and sensory neuropathy (HMSN) and tomaculous neuropathy (HNPP)

Angelo Sghirlanzoni and Davide Pareyson

Department of Neurology, National Neurological Institute 'Carlo Besta', Via Celoria 11, 20133 Milan, Italy

Summary

Hereditary motor and sensory neuropathy (HMSN) or Charcot–Marie–Tooth disease (CMT) is a heterogeneous group of neuropathies, characterized by the presence of peroneal atrophy. Transmission is autosomal dominant in most cases. Autosomal recessive or X-linked subtypes are also found. The different forms of CMT are classified according to inheritance, natural history, neurophysiological and neuropathological findings. Duplication of (or point mutations within) the chromosomal region 17p11.2–12, containing the gene for the myelin protein PMP22, causes the most frequent demyelinating form CMT1A; mutations of the protein P0 gene, mapping on chromosome 1q21.2–23, lead to a second demyelinating form, called CMT1B; mutations of the connexin-32 gene, which maps to the pericentromeric region of Xq chromosome, are responsible for the X-linked or CMTX variety; a rare recessive demyelinating form is linked to the 8q13–21.1 region; some families with the autosomal dominant axonal type (CMT2A) show linkage to the 1p35–36 region.

Autosomal dominant hereditary neuropathy with liability to pressure palsies (HNPP) is associated with a deletion of the 17p11.2–12 region, the same that is duplicated in CMT1A. Both CMT1A and HNPP are autosomal dominant, primary demyelinating neuropathies, with distinctly different clinical and histopathological features. CMT1A apparently derives from an increased dosage of the PMP22 gene, while HNPP might be the consequence of a decreased gene dosage leading to under-expression of PMP22. The CMT1A duplication and the HNPP deletion appear to result from an unequal meiotic crossing-over involving two homologous repeated sequences (CMT1A-REP) flanking the duplication/deletion monomer.

Charcot–Marie–Tooth (CMT) disease, or hereditary motor and sensory neuropathy (HMSN), has been well characterized in its essential clinical features since the first description as 'peroneal type of progressive muscular atrophy', in 1886.

Hereditary neuropathy with liability to pressure palsies (HNPP), also called tomaculous neuropathy, was originally described by De Jong (1947), in a family of coal miners in which three generations had recurrent pressure palsies doing routine work in a squatting position.

In the last few years, they have both come to the attention of neurologists and geneticists because CMT1A, the most frequent form of CMT disease, and HNPP appear to result from reciprocal DNA duplication (CMT1A) or deletion (HNPP) of the same region on chromosome 17p (17p11.2–12) (Chance et al., 1994a). The DNA rearrangement is present in most CMT1A cases (Lupski et al., 1991; Raeymaekers et al., 1991; Bellone et al., 1992) and HNPP (Chance et al., 1994a; Pareyson et al., 1996); *de novo* duplication or deletion can be responsible for sporadic cases of CMT1A or HNPP (Hoogendijk et al., 1992; Pareyson et al., 1996).

The critical 17p11.2–12 region involved in both neuropathies spans 1.5 megabases, and is likely to contain multiple genes, but a dosage effect of a single gene, encoding a myelin protein of the peripheral nerve named PMP22, appears to play a crucial role in the disease phenotype. Thus, while CMT1A apparently derives from an increased dosage of the PMP22 gene, HNPP might be the consequence of a decreased gene dosage leading to under-expression of PMP22 (Lupski et al., 1993; Chance et al., 1994a).

The autosomal dominant CMT1A phenotype was demonstrated to be due to point mutations of the PMP22 gene in occasional patients not harbouring the CMT1A duplication (Roa et al., 1993a). An HNPP patient not carrying the deletion had a frameshift mutation in one of the two PMP22 alleles (Nicholson et al., 1994).

The different forms of CMT are classified according to inheritance pattern, natural history, neurophysiological and neuropathological findings (Dyck et al., 1993). The most common subtype is the autosomal dominant, hypertrophic form: CMT1 or HMSN type I. Autosomal recessive and X-linked CMT1, however, have been reported. The axonal form, CMT2, also segregates in an autosomal dominant fashion.

Clinical features

CMT disease is a slowly progressive neuropathy beginning with atrophy of foot and leg muscles followed later by involvement of hand muscles. Affected limbs often show vasomotor abnormalities; cramps can be present. Proximal limb muscles are spared; sensory impairment is mild in most cases.

Onset of symptoms occurs within the first decade of life in 50 per cent of patients, and within the second decade in another 30 per cent.

Children are often referred to the physician because of abnormalities of gait and feet, or frequent falls due to weakness of the peroneal and tibialis anterior muscles.

Early in the disease, pes planus is more frequent than pes cavus (Feasby et al., 1992); this last deformity seems to progress with age. Atrophy of the distal leg is a prominent feature in most patients, but can be masked by thick subcutaneous fat. Reduction in muscle bulk and weakness begin first in territories supplied by long axons and later extend to districts supplied by shorter ones. The involvement of the intrinsic hand muscles, sometimes resulting in a claw hand, usually occurs late in the course of the disease, together with wasting of the distal muscles of the thigh; the latter are supplied by axons of the same length and are contemporarily involved at the same stage of disease progression.

The atrophy of the calves is virtually never so marked in childhood as to give the lower limbs the classical appearance of the 'inverted champagne bottle' or 'stork-legs' as described in adult patients. Pes cavus is the result of the imbalance between the weakened muscles in the anterior compartment and their antagonists. The toes are clawed with hyperextension of the first phalanx and hyperflexion of the others. Leg weakness and foot deformity may seriously handicap the patient because walking may be hampered by the inability to lift the forefoot.

Sensory loss is often mild or clinically undetectable, particularly in the axonal form. A glove and stocking-like distribution is the rule. Vibration sense is the most severely affected. Positive sensory signs, such as paraesthesias and burning feet, are not features of this disorder.

Reduction or loss of reflexes probably is the most constant clinical finding. In CMT1, peripheral nerves may be thickened. CMT1 and CMT2 share quite similar signs and symptoms; the two forms cannot be clinically differentiated in one particular patient.

The characteristic features of Déjérine–Sottas disease (HMSN III) should be: autosomal recessive inheritance; onset within the first 2 years of life; clinical manifestations more marked than CMT1; and more frequent enlargement of peripheral nerves than in the dominant CMT1 (Dyck *et al.*, 1993).

Neurophysiological features

The subdivision into CMT1 and CMT2 is based mainly on nerve conduction velocities (NCV), which are bimodally distributed in this population (Harding & Thomas, 1980; Sghirlanzoni *et al.*, 1990). In CMT1, NCV values less than 40 m/s are a hallmark of the disorder, being 100 per cent penetrant; slowed NCV are present even in asymptomatic patients from the age of 2–4 years (when peripheral nerve myelination is completed), and are roughly constant throughout the patient's life. Conversely, NCV are normal or slightly reduced in CMT2. Patients whose upper limb nerve NCV is >40 m/s are classified as CMT2. An inability to record conduction in the common peroneal nerve is frequent in both groups.

In HMSN III motor conduction velocity is markedly decreased to values below 12 m/s (Dyck *et al.*, 1993).

Pathological features

Abundant and multilamellated onion bulbs are typical, although not specific, alterations in CMT1.

Reduction of the density and total number of myelinated fibres is found both in CMT1 and in CMT2. In CMT2, the number of thinly myelinated fibres is increased and 'clusters' of regenerating nerve sprouts are found; poorly organized onion bulbs can rarely be seen.

In Déjérine–Sottas disease there is a marked loss of myelinated fibres with hypomyelination; very few fibres greater than 8 μn in diameter survive; onion bulbs are often large, with thin lamellae often consisting of apposed double basement membranes. The differential diagnosis between HMSN types I and III is hampered by the overlap of clinical, neurophysiological and pathological features of the two forms. In single cases, the differentiation between them may be impossible.

Killian & Kloepfer (1979) showed the genetic heterogeneity of Déjérine–Sottas disease, describing two children who met the diagnostic criteria of this disease while their parents were both affected by dominant CMT1.

A similar event has been demonstrated (Sghirlanzoni *et al.*, 1992) in a family in which the Déjérine–Sottas phenotype was determined by a homozygosity for the axonal autosomal dominant HMSN II gene.

Recessive cases of CMT1 have been reported (Dyck *et al.*, 1993). Furthermore, molecular genetic studies recently demonstrated dominant point mutations for the PMP22 and P0 genes causing the Déjérine–Sottas phenotype (Roa *et al.*, 1993b; Hayasaka *et al.*, 1993b). Consequently, we believe that Déjérine–Sottas disease is an empty box containing the most severe, sporadic, recessive or dominant forms of hereditary polyneuropathy (Sghirlanzoni *et al.*, 1994). Only molecular diagnosis will make possible accurate differentiation between the different types of demyelinating HMSN.

Genetics

CMT disease, with a prevalence of 1:2,500, is the most common inherited peripheral neuropathy, and one of the most frequent genetic disorders.

CMT1, mostly inherited as an autosomal dominant trait, may rarely show autosomal recessive or X-linked transmission.

In about 70 per cent of CMT1 patients, the disease maps to chromosome 17p11.2–12 and is called CMT1A (Wise et al., 1993). The locus for the autosomal dominant CMT1B is linked to markers on 1q21.2–23 and has been identified in the gene for the myelin protein P0 (Hayasaka et al., 1993a, c; Kulkens et al., 1993). Finally, in autosomal dominant CMT1C a third locus is linked to neither chromosome 1 nor chromosome 17 (Dyck et al., 1993).

The X-linked variant maps in the pericentromeric region of chromosome Xq and is caused by mutations in the connexin–32 gene (Bergoffen et al., 1993).

These four distinct genetic forms of CMT1 share similar phenotypes. The three identified genes causing the CMT1 subtypes encode proteins involved in compaction and maintenance of myelin (PMP22, P0) as well as in the constitution of the intercellular channels (connexin–32). It is not known whether any of these four loci is involved in the autosomal recessive form of CMT1.

In four inbred Tunisian families with 13 affected patients, there is evidence for linkage to chromosome 8q13–21.1 of a recessive form of CMT disease (Ben Othmane et al., 1993a).

CMT2 is also an autosomal dominant disease, and has been recently shown to be linked, in a minority of families, to the distal short arm of chromosome 1 (1p35–36) (Ben Othmane et al., 1993b). Autosomal dominant HNPP maps to 17p11.2–12, the same locus of CMT1A (Chance et al., 1993).

Hereditary neuropathy with liability to pressure palsies

Hereditary neuropathy with liability to pressure palsies (HNPP) is an autosomal dominant disorder characterized by recurrent mononeuropathies with electrophysiological abnormalities in nerve conduction which are more evident at common entrapment sites. Characteristic pathological changes are sausage-like myelin thickenings, commonly referred to as tomacula, in most fibres on nerve biopsy (Windebank, 1993; Marazzi et al., 1988).

In the vast majority of cases, HNPP has been associated with a submicroscopic deletion on chromosome 17p11.2–12 (Chance et al., 1993) involving the same 1.5 megabase interval that is duplicated in CMT1A (Lupski et al., 1991) and that includes the PMP22 gene (Patel et al., 1992). According to the current working hypothesis, the CMT1A duplication and the HNPP deletion represent the two reciprocal recombination products of an unequal meiotic cross-over involving two homologous repeated sequences (CMT1A-REP) which flank the duplication/deletion monomer (Pentao et al., 1992; Lupski et al., 1993; Chance et al., 1994a). HNPP families and sporadic cases showing evidence of deletion of this chromosomal region have been reported from different countries (Le Guern et al., 1994; Mariman et al., 1994; Reisecker et al., 1994; Verhalle et al., 1994; Lorenzetti et al., 1995). In some HNPP families, however, the deletion was not found (Mariman et al., 1994); in one case, a frameshift mutation in a PMP22 allele was demonstrated, which would result in premature termination of PMP22 (Nicholson et al., 1994).

In our series of 39 HNPP patients from 16 unrelated families carrying the deletion, extensive clinical and electrophysiological analysis reveal phenotypic heterogeneity despite genotypic homogeneity (Pareyson et al., 1996). The expression variability may be observed both within and among families. The spectrum of phenotypic expression of deleted HNPP appears to be broader than previously thought. Therefore, on clinical grounds, diagnosis of isolated cases and identification of affected relatives may prove to be difficult. Two-thirds of our patients had had at least one episode of acute mononeuropathy, often involving nerve territories of the upper limbs (36 per cent) or brachial plexus (31 per cent); however, 41 per cent of affected individuals were unaware of their disease, and 25 per cent were almost or completely asymptomatic; 33 per cent of patients complained of chronic symptoms such as paraesthesias, muscle cramps, or exercise-induced myalgias.

The pattern and severity of electrophysiological abnormalities differed considerably among affected subjects, ranging from conduction abnormalities localized at common entrapment sites to diffuse slowing of nerve conduction, usually more evident at entrapment sites; rarely, patients may show pre-eminent proximal conduction slowing.

It is likely that the same pathogenetic mechanism underlies both the mononeuropathy and the plexopathy, the only difference being the site of peripheral involvement. Plexopathy and mononeuropathy in subsequent episodes in the same patient and in different members of the same family can be observed. Brachial plexopathy is known to occur in HNPP, sometimes as the only clinical manifestation (Bosch *et al.*, 1980; Martinelli *et al.*, 1989). HNPP plexopathy is clearly distinguished from hereditary neuralgic amyotrophy (HNA) because of differing precipitating events and the absence of pain (Windebank, 1993). Furthermore, evidence that the two disorders are genetically distinct has been recently provided (Chance *et al.*, 1994b; Gouider *et al.*, 1994). Plexus cord compression in the supraclavicular region, stretching, and friction against surrounding structures may play a role in the pathogenesis of plexopathy.

A few patients, often with long-lasting symptoms, can show a picture of polyneuropathy, with superimposed mononeuropathies. At first sight, these patients could be misdiagnosed as being affected with Charcot–Marie–Tooth disease. A chronic course of tomaculous neuropathy mimicking CMT disease has also been reported (Barbieri *et al.*, 1990). Notably, pes cavus is frequent in HNPP (38 per cent of our cases).

HNPP is often benign; the onset of symptoms ranges between 8 and 64 years (mean 26.5), and in 50 per cent of symptomatic patients occurs within the second decade of life.

In patients unaware of their peripheral nerve disorder, whilst diagnosis could not always be made on clinical grounds alone, electrophysiological examination was always diagnostic and consistent with genetic data, provided that conduction slowing at entrapment sites was specifically investigated. Conduction abnormalities at entrapment sites are frequently found and proved to be the most reliable finding for diagnosis: 87.5 per cent of our patients showed conduction slowing in at least one site. Susceptibility of nerves to compression appears to be the common mechanism underlying all the different HNPP phenotypes, the clinical variability being highly influenced by the occurrence of exogenous factors. Variability may also reflect the molecular mechanism of HNPP, as the reduced PMP22 gene dosage might enhance the influence of modifier genes, if any, or environmental effects.

There are some different methods to demonstrate the HNPP deletion or the CMT1A duplication. We employed three methods (Lorenzetti *et al.*, 1995): (1) typization of families with polymorphic markers mapping within the deleted region (RM11-GT microsatellite by PCR; RLFP VAW409R3a, VAW412R3 and EW401, by Southern blot) demonstrating a lack of allelic transmission from affected parents to affected offspring; (2) Southern blot with *EcoRI*-digested DNA employing a 1.8 kb *EcoRI* fragment cloned from the pNEA102 probe which recognizes the CMT1A-REP: increased hybridization intensity signal of the 6.0 kb fragment (corresponding to the distal CMT1A-REP) relative to the 7.8 kb fragment (corresponding to the proximal CMT1A-REP) provides evidence of the loss of one CMT1A-REP in the HNPP deleted chromosome; (3) pulsed field gel electrophoresis (PFGE) analysis of the HNPP *Sac*II junction fragments. Following PFGE of *Sac*II-digested genomic DNA and Southern transfer, DNA is hybridized with probe pNEA101 which maps to the proximal CMT1A-REP element. Because of the differential methylation of the *Sac*II site proximal to the duplication/deletion region, two HNPP junction fragments, of 770 kb or 820 kb, can be detected (Lorenzetti et al., 1995).

PFGE appears to be the first-choice method for the molecular diagnosis of HNPP, because it allows, with a single experiment, direct and clear-cut demonstration of both the HNPP deletion and the CMT1A duplication in single patients, thus eliminating the need for segregation analysis of families (Lupski et al., 1993).

In our series, all the cases diagnosed as HNPP on clinical and neuropathological grounds carried the deletion. Different findings were reported by Mariman et al. (1994), with seven out of 22 HNPP families having no evidence of the deletion.

If the unequal crossing-over hypothesis is correct, one should expect a prevalence of HNPP close to that of CMT1A (about 1:5000), unless a negative selection against the deleted chromosome is present. It is conceivable that the actual frequency of HNPP is currently underestimated and that many cases are not recognized. Possible reasons are misdiagnosis, difficulties in assessing inheritance, and benignity of the neuropathy.

This is the reason why the molecular demonstration of the deletion is going to become a key tool in the differential diagnosis of peripheral neuropathies and plexopathies.

Differential diagnosis

Any clinician involved in the care of patients with peripheral neuropathy experienced the diagnostic difficulties in distinguishing HMSN I and HMSN III from other inherited demyelinating neuropathies. A general criterion is that CMT, as well as HNPP, are strictly limited to the peripheral nervous system (PNS) (PMP22 and P0 are PNS proteins), and these diseases can be excluded in all cases of central nervous system (CNS) involvement. Refsum's disease has a recognized and identifiable defect of phytanic acid metabolism.

In sporadic cases, difficulties also arise in the differential diagnosis between CMT1 or Déjérine–Sottas disease and chronic inflammatory demyelinating polyradiculoneuropathies (CIDP). On taking a careful history, CIDP almost always shows an episodic or fluctuating course; at examination, CIDP patients often show signs of involvement of both proximal and distal muscle groups; electrophysiological findings are characterized by nonhomogeneous conduction slowing and blocks. Although biopsy changes can be similar to HMSN I, lymphocytes and macrophages are usually evident.

The clinical picture of CMT in childhood is of peroneal muscular atrophy and distal weakness. Conduction slowing, in demyelinating CMT forms, is always highly symmetrical, diffuse and homogeneous (without focal slowing) along both the proximal and distal segments of motor and sensory nerves (Scaioli et al., 1992).

In HNPP, nerve conduction velocities range from normal to diffusely slowed, usually in an asymmetric and nonhomogeneous pattern. Conduction abnormalities are more evident at common entrapment sites. Proximal slowing, as revealed by prolonged F-latencies, may be the pre-eminent abnormality in a minority of HNPP patients. The electrophysiological differential diagnosis between HNPP and chronic inflammatory demyelinating polyradiculoneuropathy and motor neuropathy with multifocal conduction blocks largely relies on a different clinical course as well as on the distribution of the focal slowing, which is randomly scattered in these diseases. Nerve biopsies are more sensitive than specific in HNPP diagnosis. Although their presence is deemed to be necessary for diagnosis, tomacula (focal thickenings of the myelin sheath) have also been described in other neuropathies, either inherited or acquired. Thus, the specificity of tomacula for diagnosis of HNPP relies more on their number than on their mere presence. The indication for nerve biopsy in HNPP patients has now been overcome by the non-invasive molecular genetic diagnosis, but is still valid in non-deleted patients with evidence of multiple entrapments.

Myopathies usually affect proximal muscles. In the quite rare distal myopathies and in some cases of mitochondrial myopathies, the clinical picture may resemble peroneal muscular atrophy, but nerve conduction studies are normal; EMG and muscle biopsy show characteristic changes.

There is a number of patients presenting with pes cavus in whom no neuromuscular disorder can be documented. True idiopathic pes cavus is often familial. It should be diagnosed only after detailed investigations have ruled out other diagnostic alternatives.

Acknowledgement

This research was supported by Telethon–Italia grant nos. 560 and 924 to Angelo Sghirlanzoni.

References

Barbieri, F., Santangelo, R., Crisci, C., Ragno, M., Perretti, A. & Santoro, L. (1990): A family with tomaculous neuropathy mimicking Charcot–Marie–Tooth disease. *Clin. Neurol. Neurosurg.* **92,** 289–294.

Bellone, E., Mandich, P., Mancardi, G.L., Schenone, A., Uccelli, A., Abbruzzese, M., Sghirlanzoni, A., Pareyson, D. & Ajmar, F. (1992): Charcot–Marie–Tooth (CMT) 1a duplication at 17p11.2 in Italian families. *J. Med. Genet.* **29,** 492–493.

Ben Othmane, K., Hentati, F., Lennon, F., Ben Hamida, C., Blel, S., Roses, A. D., Pericak-Vance, M.A., Ben Hamida, M. & Vance, J.M. (1993a): Linkage of a locus (CMT4A) for autosomal recessive Charcot–Marie–Tooth disease to chromosome 8q. *Hum. Molec. Genet.* **2,** 1625–1628.

Ben Othmane, K., Middleton, L.T., Loprest, L.J., Wilkinson, K.M., Lennon, F., Rozear, M.P., Stajich, J.M., Gaskell, P.C., Roses, A.D., Pericak-Vance, M. A. & Vance, J.M. (1993b): Localization of a gene (CMT2A) for autosomal dominant Charcot–Marie–Tooth disease type 2 to chromosome 1p and evidence of genetic heterogeneity. *Genomics* **17,** 370–375.

Bergoffen, J., Scherer, S.S., Wang, S., Oronzi Scott, M., Bone, L.J., Paul, D.L., Chen, K., Lensch, M.W., Chance, P.F. & Fischbeck, K.H. (1993): Connexin mutations in X-linked Charcot–Marie–Tooth disease. *Science* **262,** 2039–2042.

Bosch, E.P., Chui, H.C., Martin, M.A. & Cancilla, P.A. (1980): Brachial plexus involvement in familial pressure-sensitive neuropathy: electrophysiological and morphological findings. *Ann. Neurol.* **8,** 620–624.

Chance, P.F., Alderson, M.K., Leppig, K.A., Lensch, M.W., Matsunami, N., Smith, B., Swanson, P.D., Odelberg, S.J., Disteche, C.M. & Bird, T.D. (1993): DNA deletion associated with hereditary neuropathy with liability to pressure palsies. *Cell* **72,** 143–151.

Chance, P.F., Abbas, N., Lensch, M.W., Pentao, L., Roa, B.B., Patel, P.I. & Lupski, J.R. (1994a): Two autosomal dominant neuropathies result from reciprocal DNA duplication/deletion of a region on chromosome 17. *Hum. Mol. Genet.* **3,** 223–228.

Chance, P.F., Lensch, M.W., Lipe, H., Brown, R.H. Sr., Brown, R.H. Jr. & Bird, T.D. (1994b): Hereditary neuralgic amyotrophy and hereditary neuropathy with liability to pressure palsies: two distinct genetic disorders. *Neurology* **44,** 2253–2257.

De Jong, J.G.I. (1947): Over families met hereditaire dispositie tot het optreden van neuritiden gecorreleerd met migraine. *Psychiatr. Neurol. Bull.* **50,** 60–76.

Dyck, P.J., Chance, P., Lebo, R. & Carney, J.A. (1993): Hereditary motor and sensory neuropathies. In: *Peripheral neuropathy,* eds. P.J. Dyck, P.K. Thomas, J.W. Griffin, P.A. Low & J.F. Poduslo, pp.1094–1136. 3rd ed. Philadelphia: W.B. Saunders.

Feasby, T.E., Hahn, A.F., Bolton, C.F., Brown, W.F. & Koopman, W.J. (1992): Detection of hereditary motor sensory neuropathy type I in childhood. *J. Neurol. Neurosurg. Psychiatry* **55,** 895–897.

Gouider, R., Le Guern, E., Emile, J., Tardieu, S., Cabon, F., Samid, M., Weissenbach, J., Agid, Y., Bouche, P. & Brice, A. (1994): Hereditary neuralgic amyotrophy and hereditary neuropathy with pressure palsies: two distinct clinical, electrophysiologic, and genetic entities. *Neurology* **44,** 2250–2252.

Harding, A.E. & Thomas, P.K. (1980): The clinical features of hereditary motor and sensory neuropathy types I and II. *Brain* **103,** 259–280.

Hayasaka, K., Himoro, M., Sato, W., Takada, G., Uyemura, K., Shimizu, N., Bird, T.D., Conneally, P.M. & Chance, P.F. (1993a): Charcot–Marie–Tooth neuropathy type 1B is associated with mutations of the myelin P0 gene. *Nature Genet.* **5**, 31–34.

Hayasaka, K., Himoro, M., Sawaishi, Y., Nanao, K., Takahashi, T., Takada, G., Nicholson, G.A., Ouvrier, R.A. & Tachi, N. (1993b): De novo mutation of the myelin P0 gene in Dejerine–Sottas disease (hereditary motor and sensory neuropathy type III). *Nature Genet.* **5**, 266–268.

Hayasaka, K., Takada, G. & Ionasescu, V. (1993c): Mutation of the myelin P0 gene in Charcot–Marie–Tooth neuropathy type 1B. *Hum. Molec. Genet.* **2**, 1369–1371.

Hoogendijk, J.E,, Hensels, G.W., Gabreels-Festen, A.A.W.M., Gabreels, F.J.M., Janssen, E.A.M., De Jonghe, P., Martin, J-J., Van Broeckhoven, C., Valentijn, L.J., Baas, F., De Visser, M. & Bolhuis, P.A. (1992): *De novo* mutation in hereditary motor and sensory neuropathy type 1. *Lancet* **339**, 1081–1082.

Killian, J.M. & Kloepfer, H.W. (1979): Homozygous expression of a dominant gene for Charcot–Marie–Tooth neuropathy. *Ann. Neurol.* **5**, 515–522.

Kulkens, T., Bolhuis, P.A., Wolterman, R.A., Kemp, S., te Nijenhuis, S., Valentijn, L.J., Hensel, G.W., Jennekens, F.G.I., De Visser, M., Hoogendijk, J.E., & Baas, F. (1993): Deletion of the serine 34 codon from the major peripheral myelin protein P0 gene in Charcot–Marie–Tooth disease type 1B. *Nature Genet.* **5**, 35–39.

Le Guern, E., Sturtz, F., Gugenheim, M., Gouider, R., Bonnebouche, C., Ravisé, N., Gonnaud, P-M., Tardieu, S., Bouche, P., Chazot, G., Agid, Y., Vanderberghe, A. & Brice, A. (1994): Detection of deletion within 17p11.2 in 7 French families with hereditary neuropathy with liability to pressure palsies (HNPP). *Cytogenet. Cell. Genet.* **65**, 261–264.

Lorenzetti, D., Pareyson, D., Sghirlanzoni, A., Roa, B.B., Abbas, N.E., Pandolfo, M., Di Donato, S. & Lupski, J.R. (1995): A 1.5 Md deletion in 17p11.2-p12 is frequently observed in Italian families with hereditary neuropathy with liability to pressure palsies. *Am. J. Hum. Genet.* **56**, 91–98.

Lupski, J.R., Montes de Oca-Luna, R., Slaugenhaupt, S., Pentao, L., Guzzetta, V., Trask, B.J., Saucedo-Cardenas, O., Barker, D.F., Killian, J.M., Garcia, C.A., Chakravarti, A. & Patel, P.I. (1991): DNA duplication associated with Charcot–Marie–Tooth disease type 1A. *Cell* **66**, 219–232.

Lupski, J.R., Chance, P.F. & Garcia, C.A. (1993): Inherited primary peripheral neuropathies. Molecular genetics and clinical implications of CMT1A and HNPP. *JAMA* **270**, 2326–2330.

Marazzi, R., Pareyson, D., Scaioli, V., Corbo, M., Boiardi, A., Chiodelli, G. & Sghirlanzoni, A. (1988): Recurrent familial neuropathy due to liability to pressure palsies. *Ital. J. Neurol. Sci.* **9**, 355–363.

Mariman, E.C.M., Gabreels-Festen, A.A.W.M., van Beersum, S.E.C., Valentijn, L.J., Baas, F., Bolhuis, P.A., Jongen, P.J.H., Ropers, H.H. & Gabreels, F.J.M. (1994): Prevalence of the 1.5-Mb 17p deletion in families with hereditary neuropathy with liability to pressure palsies. *Ann. Neurol.* **36**, 650–655.

Martinelli, P., Fabbri, R., Moretto, G., Gabellini, A.S., D'Alessandro, R. & Rizzuto, N. (1989): Recurrent familial brachial plexus palsies as the only clinical expression of 'tomaculous' neuropathy. *Eur. Neurol.* **29**, 61–66.

Nicholson, G.A., Valentijn, L.J., Cherryson, A.K., Kennerson, M.L., Bragg, T.L., DeKroon, R.M., Ross, D.A., Pollard, J.D., McLeod, J.G., Bolhuis, P.A. & Baas, F. (1994): A frame shift mutation in the PMP-22 gene in hereditary neuropathy with liability to pressure palsies. *Nature Genet.* **6**, 263–266.

Pareyson, D., Scaioli, V., Taroni, F., Botti, S., Lorenzetti, D., Solari, A., Ciano, C. & Sghirlanzoni, A. (1996): Phenotypic heterogeneity in hereditary neuropathy with liability to pressure palsies associated with chromosome 17p11. 1–12 deletion. *Neurology* **46**, 1133–1137.

Patel, P.I., Roa, B.B., Welcher, A.A., Schoener-Scott, R., Trask, B.J., Pentao, L., Snipes, G.J., Garcia, C.A., Francke, U., Shooter, E.M., Lupski, J.R. & Suter, U. (1992): The gene for peripheral myelin protein PMP-22 is a candidate for Charcot–Marie–Tooth disease type 1A. *Nature Genet.* **1**, 157–165.

Pentao, L., Wise, C.A., Chinault, A.C., Patel, P.I. & Lupski J.R. (1992): Charcot–Marie–Tooth type 1A duplication appears to arise from recombination at repeat sequences flanking the 1.5 Mb monomer unit. *Nature Genet.* **2**, 292–300.

Raeymaekers, P., Timmerman, V., Nelis, E., De Jonghe, P., Hoogendijk, J.E., Baas, F., Barker, D.F., Martin, J.J., De Visser, M., Bolhuis P.A. & Van Broeckhoven, C. (1991): Duplication in chromosome 17p11.2 in Charcot–Marie–Tooth neuropathy type 1a (CMT 1a). *Neuromusc. Dis.* **1**, 93–97.

Reisecker, F., Leblhuber, F., Lexner, R., Radner, G., Rosenkranz, W. & Wagner, K. (1994): A sporadic form of hereditary neuropathy with liability to pressure palsies: clinical, electrodiagnostic, and molecular genetic findings. *Neurology* **44**, 753–755.

Roa, B.B., Garcia, C.A., Suter, U., Kulpa, D.A., Wise, C.A., Mueller, J., Welcher, A.A., Snipes, G.J., Shooter, E.M., Patel, P.I. & Lupski, J.R. (1993a): Charcot–Marie–Tooth disease type 1A. Association with a spontaneous point mutation in the PMP22 gene. *N. Engl. J. Med.* **329**, 96–101.

Roa, B.B., Dyck, P.J., Marks, H.G., Chance, P.F. & Lupski, J.R. (1993b): Dejerine–Sottas syndrome associated with point mutation in the peripheral myelin protein 22 (PMP22) gene. *Nature Genet.* **5**, 269–273.

Scaioli, V., Pareyson, D., Avanzini, G. & Sghirlanzoni, A. (1992): F-response, somatosensory and brainstem auditory evoked potential studies in HMSN type I and II. *J. Neurol. Neurosurg. Psychiatry* **55**, 1027–1031.

Sghirlanzoni, A., Pareyson, D., Scaioli, V., Marazzi, R. & Pacini, L. (1990): Hereditary motor and sensory neuropathy type I and type II. *Ital. J. Neurol. Sci.* **11**, 471–479.

Sghirlanzoni, A., Pareyson, D., Balestrini, M.R., Bellone, E., Berta, E., Ciano, C., Mandich, P. & Marazzi, R. (1992): HMSN III phenotype due to homozygous expression of a dominant HMSN II gene. *Neurology* **42**, 2201–2203.

Sghirlanzoni, A., Pareyson, D., Marazzi, R., Cavaletti, G., Bellone, E., Mandich, P., Balestrini, M.R. & Riva, D. (1994): Homozygous hypertrophic hereditary motor and sensory neuropathies. *Ital. J. Neurol. Sci.* **15**, 5–14.

Verhalle, D., Lofgren, A., Nelis, E., Dehaene, I., Theys, P., Lammens, M., Dom, R., Van Broeckhoven, C. & Robberecht, W. (1994): Deletion in CMT1A locus on chromosome 17p11.2 in hereditary neuropathy with liability to pressure palsies. *Ann. Neurol.* **35**, 704–708.

Windebank, A.J. (1993): Inherited recurrent focal neuropathies. In: *Peripheral neuropathy*, 3rd edn., eds. P.J. Dyck, P.K. Thomas, J.W. Griffin, P.A. Low & J.F. Poduslo, pp. 1137–1148. Philadelphia: W.B. Saunders.

Wise, C.A., Garcia, C.A., Davis, S.N., Heju, Z., Pentao, L., Patel, P.I. & Lupski, J.R. (1993): Molecular analyses of unrelated Charcot–Marie–Tooth (CMT) disease patients suggest a high frequency of the CMT1A duplication. *Am. J. Hum. Genet.* **53**, 853–863.

Chapter 8

Spinal muscular atrophy: history and personal observations

Giovanni Lanzi, Angela Berardinelli and Andrea Gemma

Department of Child Neuropsychiatry, C. Mondino Institute, University of Pavia, Via Palestro 3, 27100 Pavia, Italy

Summary

The authors review quickly the historical descriptions of proximal spinal muscular atrophies (SMA), stressing especially the problems of classification and the unanswered questions regarding the pathogenesis and wide clinical variability. They then describe their personal observations about groups of patients affected by SMA types I, II and III, who have been followed up by t he authors, and underline the most important clinical problems for each type.

A long time has passed since the first clinical reports of spinal muscular atrophy (SMA) were published by Werdnig (1891) and Hoffman (1893), and it is striking how even these early authors clearly described the main characteristics of the disease, such as the symptomatology, inheritance and its progression.

The clinical aspects of SMA have been better defined since 1954, thanks to the work of Kugelberg & Welander (1954), which showed how the age of onset could vary and related the different symptomatologies to it.

In recent years there has been much discussion as to whether the cases described by Werdnig and Hoffman and those described by Kugelberg & Welander could be referred to the same pathology. This problem now seems to be solved, and the proximal types of SMA at least are all due to the same genetic defect (MacKenzie et al., 1994; Munsat et al., 1990; Winsor et al., 1971).

In this paper we shall discuss the proximal types of SMA.

Recent advances

In recent months two separate study groups, based in France (Lefebvre, 1995) and in Canada (Roy et al., 1995) have discussed two different genes, mapped in the 5q 13.1 region, which are responsible for the three classical, proximal types of SMA.

The French group has mapped a 20 kb gene that codes for a new 294 amino acid protein. The telomeric region of this gene was interrupted in 226 of the 229 patients they studied, and in the remaining three patients there was a point mutation or a small deletion in the same region.

The coding region has been denominated the 'SMN-gene' (survival motor neuron gene). No relation has been found between the genotype and the phenotype.

The Canadian group has identified another gene, in the same 5q 13.1 region, which codes for the protein that inhibits apoptosis. Apoptosis is a programmed cell death which is hystologically characterised by cellular swelling and chromatolysis.

The central role of apoptosis in normal embryogenesis has been understood during the last two decades (Oppenheim, 1991; Sarnat, 1992; Fidzianska et al., 1990). In SMA there is probably a pathological reactivation or a failure to disactivate apoptosis.

The relation between the two genes that have been mapped is still to be worked out, but it is probably the cause of SMA and of their clinical heterogeneity (Lefebvre, 1995; Roy et al., 1995).

Unanswered questions

The pathogenesis and clinical heterogeneity of SMA are two of the many problems that are still unsolved, which regard the genetic biochemical mechanism which is responsible for the disease. Furthermore, the most important symptoms and signs for prognosis are still to be defined and the issue of the interpretation of those cases which do not perfectly fit present classifications has not yet been resolved (Appelbaum et al., 1992; Benady, 1978; Brustowicz et al., 1991, 1993; Davies et al., 1991; Davies & Munsat, 1995; Dubowitz, 1991; Emery et al., 1976; Fidzianska et al., 1990; Gordon, 1991; Greensmith & Vrabova, 1995; Hausmanowa-Petrusewicz, 1991; Henderson et al., 1993; Munsat et al., 1990 Munsat & Davies, 1992).

All this explains the extent of genetic research (Brzustowicz et al., 1991, 1993; Davies et al., 1991; Emery, 1991; Gennarelli et al., 1992; Henderson et al., 1993; Kleyn & Gilliam, 1993; La Spada et al., 1992; Lusakowska et al., 1994; MacKenzie et al., 1994; Melki, 1991; Merette et al., 1994; Munsat et al., 1990; Rietschel et al., 1992; Simard et al., 1992) and also clinical research throughout the world in recent years.

We have chosen proximal SMA as the subject of our paper, as this group is quite homogeneous and much more frequent than the so-called distal SMA, and we have quite long experience of therapeutic clinical aspects of these disease (Lanzi et al., 1977, 1993; Balottin et al., 1991).

We shall describe our patients and attempt to relate them to current problems, such as classification, the presence of prognostic indices (if any) and clinical course.

We shall leave the specific problem of pathogenesis to the geneticists, though we shall suggest what, in our opinion, are the most promising aspects for study.

Classification

The classification of proximal SMA has been a hotly debated problem for many years, and is of relevance for both clinical practice and research. Indeed any classification system expresses the state of our knowledge concerning a particular pathology, but is also the basis for deciding the diagnosis and prognosis of patients. As far as SMA is concerned many of these problems are still unclear.

Although in recent years genetic analysis has become progressively more important for diagnosis, an effective classification system is of great use to clinicians and could indeed be based on co-operation between clinicians and geneticists.

History of the classification system

In 1961 Byers & Benker proposed a classification which stressed the relation between age at onset, clinical variability and prognosis.

In 1964 Dubowitz classified SMA, basing his classification on the maximum motor ability that the patient had had, though he also confirmed the importance of age at onset in his classification.

Hausmanowa-Petrusewicz then classified SMA on the basis of ambulatory ability through time (Hausmanowa-Petrusewicz, 1991; Hausmanowa-Petrusewicz et al., 1992).

Finally, in 1989, Grimm and Fischbeck each proposed classifications for SMA, but neither fits well, the former being too dogmatic, the latter too confused.

At present the most commonly used classification system is that proposed by Dubowitz. Although it is not 'perfect', and does not fit all the cases that may be observed, it is very clear and easy to use.

Table 1. Definitions of SMA

Spinal muscular atrophy (SMA)

The spinal musclar atrophies are a group of genetically determined disorders in which there is degeneration of the anterior horn cells of the spinal cord and associated muscle weakness, which is usually symmetrical, affects the legs more than the arms and the proximal muscles more than the distal muscles. Distinct clinical syndromes can be defined on the basis of varying severity. A simple and practical clinical classification is based on the ability of the child to sit unaided and to stand and walk unaided.
1. Severe: unable to sit unsupported
2. Intermediate: able to sit unsuported: unable to stand or walk unaided
3. Mild: able to stand and walk unaided

Note that this is an arbitrary subdivision and there is varying severity within each group and that the groups merge into each other.

Severe SMA (Werdnig–Hoffmann disease)

Definition
An autosomal recessive disorder of early infancy with severe axial and limb weakness due to degeneration of the anterior horn cells of the spinal cord
Age of onset
In utero or within the first few months of life
Presenting symptoms
Hypotonia and weakness
Sucking and swallowing difficulty
Respiratory problems
Cardinal clinical signs
Severe limb and axial weakness; frog posture
Marked hypotonia
Poor head control
Diaphragmatic breathing, costal recession
Bell-shaped chest
Internal rotation of arms: jug-handle posture
Normal facial movements
Absent tendon movements
Weak cry
Associated features
Normal intellectual development

Course and prognosis
Despite severity, weakness usually non-progressive
Prone to respiratory infections
Prognosis poor; majority die of pneumonia in first year, most within 3 years
Investigations
CK: normal
Motor nerve conduction velocity normal or reduced; poor motor action potential
Ultrasonography: normal or increased echo plus atrophy of muscle
EMG: features of denervation
Muscle biopsy
Large group atrophy plus isolated or clusters of large fibres (uniformly type 1); early cases may show minimal changes – prepathological
Genetics
Autosomal recessive; gene location on chromosome 5q13.1.
Management
Pharyngeal suction if bulbar weakness present
Spinal brace in less severe cases to maintain sitting posture
Supportive treatment of pneumonia

By kind permission of Professor Dubowitz.

Dubowitz has recently (1995) proposed a numerical scoring system with decimal subdivisions, to provide a better classification of the clinical situation of individual patients (the range is from 1.0 to 3.9, with 4.0 as the 'NORMAL' score). So far cases have usually been classified on the basis of Dubowitz's previous classification, which subdivides proximal SMA into three types (Table 1).

Personal observations

SMA I

We have studied a group of 27 patients affected by SMA I (12 males and 15 females), referred for diagnosis to our Department between 1974 and 1995. The age at the first evaluation ranged from the first days of life to 8 months.

Inclusion criteria

Diagnosis was based on clinical assessment and histopathological analysis of muscle biopsy, according to Dubowitz's criteria (see Table 1) (Dubowitz, 1989).

None presented neurological problems in their kin groups or signs of CNS involvement, and no problems were reported during pregnancy.

Clinical description

Age at onset was:

    0–1 month in 8 cases (four males and four females)
    1–3 months in 16 cases (six males and ten females)
    3–6 months in 3 cases (two males and one female).

In two cases the onset of disease could be related to specific events – in one to the administration of antipolio vaccine (Sabin), and in the other to exanthem subitum.

Twenty-six of the 27 patients have undergone at least one clinical assessment in our department. The other patient was the sister of one of our patients, and we gained our information from her parents, as her clinical state was critical and she lived a great distance away.

At the time of our neurological assessment, all the children presented severe hypotonia and generalized muscle weakness, with the absence of deep tendon reflexes, and sparing of facial muscles. Their position was frog-like, and they had a barrel chest with superficial and diaphragmatic breathing.

The only motor abilities were a slow and difficult rotation of the head on the bed and flexion–extension of feet and hands. Only three patients could raise their upper limbs.

In two cases there was a mild tightness of the hips and knees. Three patients were assessed two or three times over a 2–3 month period; the others had just one clinical evaluation and we then had further information from the parents.

We did not find any significant variation through time in the three patients with more than one evaluation and their parents' reports confirmed this picture. They reported that the children were quite stable until they suddenly worsened and died as a result of respiratory failure.

Four cases were familial (two children per parent couple). We shall summarize our information on the clinical progression of 22 of the 27 patients.

Nineteen children died (eight males and 11 females); 15 in the first year of life and four after the first year of life (5½ years, 17 months, 15 months, and 14 months). Three children are still alive: two boys, of whom one is just 4½ months old, and the other is 4 years old and has been using a positive pressure mechanical ventilator (BiPAP) for 45 min per day for a year; and one girl, who is 3 years old and has been using a mechanical ventilator (BIRD) for a year (Cerveri et al., 1993; Manni et al., 1993).

Both ventilated children frequently present chest infections. They can raise their forearms and use their hands, but cannot reach their mouths. For both, disease onset was in the first months of life. Twenty-six of the 27 patients were very alert (the other also had Down's syndrome). Two baby girls, born to two couples of healthy, non-consanguineous parents, had a very similar clinical course: onset was between the first and second month of life, there was severe generalized respiratory involvement and death was in the first year of life due to respiratory failure.

Conclusions

Our SMA I cases fit those described by other workers, e.g. Thomas & Dubowitz (1994).

From a clinical point of view, patients affected by SMA I seem to be a very homogeneous group, probably because their symptoms are extremely severe, and the prognosis (death) is in most cases closely related to age of onset.

Indeed in the only two patients who survived more than 1 year, onset was between the fourth and fifth month of life. These two patients are an exception to the mean survival time. Similar cases have been described by other workers, and it would be important to investigate the genetic aspects of such cases.

Their longer survival may be related to their better chest development, i.e. the earlier the onset, the more the respiratory muscles are affected, and the less the chest mobility and lung maturation. This hypothesis has also been proposed by Thomas & Dubowitz (1994).

Personal observations

SMA II

Our SMA II cases were observed in various other Italian centres as well as our own: the Child Neuropsychiatry Departments at Genoa and Rome and the Neurological Clinics at Padua and Bari.

Clinical description

We have gathered information on 60 patients, 30 males and 30 females. The mean age at the first clinical evaluation was 6 years 6 months (range: 10 months–24 years). The mean age at onset was 6–7 months, slightly later for males (7.2) than for females (6.1). In 25 cases, the first symptoms appeared at the end of the first semester of life, in 35 cases later.

Inclusion criteria

All our patients attained the ability to sit independently, and for this reason have been defined as type II SMA. For many, however, onset was earlier than would be supposed from the classification. We were of course unable to check age at onset directly, having to rely on information from the mothers, but their reports seemed very reliable.

As we have mentioned, the classification system is open to refinement, and it may be noted that it is not always possible to find a perfect correlation between attaining the ability to sit independently and the onset of the disease in the second semester of life.

We believe that this is understandable, in as much as SMA II is not as severe a disease as type I, and so patients are able to achieve some degree of motor ability, even after the appearance of the first symptoms (Iannacone et al., 1993).

Active foetal movements were reported as being on time in 80 per cent of cases, late in 12 per cent, and reduced in 8 per cent. One-third of our patients presented a reduction of spontaneous motility and mild hypotonia at birth, and in 57 per cent motor development was slightly delayed. In our opinion, this slight delay in motor development and hypotonia at birth are of great interest because they imply that the disease can begin very early in life, even though it only becomes evident in the ensuing months. This hypothesis needs confirmation with further data.

It is probably now possible to have more detailed information about newborns and infants and we hope to succeed in confirming our hypothesis or to define the question better.

Table 2. Intermediate SMA

Definition	**Course and prognosis**
An autosomal recessive disorder characterized by weakness, predominantly of the legs, with ability to sit unsupported but not to stand, due to degeneration of the anterior horn cells of the spinal cord	Muscle weakness usually static and non-progressive; may show functional improvement: some may have increasing weakness or disability over long period or during growth spurt or if putting on weight Long-term prognosis dependent on respiratory function
Age of onset	
Usually between 6 and 12 months	
Presenting symptoms	**Investigations**
Weakness of legs	CK: normal or moderately elevated
Inability to stand or walk	Ultrasonography: characteristic picture of increased echo in muscle plus muscle atrophy and increased subcutaneous space
Cardinal clinical signs	
Symmetrical weakness of legs, predominantly proximal Able to sit unsupported but unable to stand or take full weight on legs	ECG: normal complexes: characteristic baseline EMG: evidence of denervation and re-innervation
Fasciculation of tongue (about 70 per cent)	**Muscle biopsy**
Tremor of hands	Characteristic pattern of large group atrophy plus variable clusters of enlarged fibres, uniformly or predominantly type 1
Tendon jerks absent or diminished	
Facial muscles spared	
Associated features	**Genetics**
Scoliosis	Autosomal recessive; gene location on chromosome 5q13.1
Normal or advanced intellect	
Variable intercostal weakness and respiratory problems	Alleles of one gene to account for varying severities of SMA, or dual genes or separate genes
Hypotonia and excessive joint laxity, especially hands and feet	**Management**
	Prevention of scoliosis by early bracing
	Treatment of scoliosis by spinal braces or surgery
	Early achievement of standing posture in standing frame or calipers
	Promotion of ambulation by appropriate orthoses

By kind permission of Professor Dubowitz.

Follow-up

Most (50/60) were sporadic cases; only 10 were familial (six different families). Different types of SMA were present in two families: (1) a boy with type I/II SMA and his sister with type III SMA; (2) two sisters, one with type II and the other type III SMA. There was good correlation between age at onset and clinical progression in the other families.

Onset of the disease was related to chest infections in eight patients, and in two others to exanthematic diseases. These are usually considered to be pure coincidence. We have followed up seven of these patients for at least 6 years in our clinic.

They were evaluated on the basis of three clinical parameters included in our research protocol: the ability to roll, motor functions of lower limbs, and scoliosis.

All our cases worsened during follow up. Six of these children (two boys and four girls) died aged between 8 and 23 years. Two of them were able to attain new motor abilities, even though these were late and transient. This transient motor ability is particularly shown by the rolling function.

We have also found the possibility for improvement in neurological abilities in other patients who were not included in this group because their follow-up period was too short. This may be explained by the fact that if the disease is not too severe at the beginning, it may not stop neurological development, which is very strong in the first years of life.

It is also worth noting that four out of seven patients had such severe respiratory failure that they needed mechanical ventilators (BiPAP-ST/D, BIRD) (Cerveri *et al.*, 1993; Manni *et al.*, 1993; Wang *et al.*, 1994).

SMA III

We again used Dubowitz's criteria for the definition of this group (see Table 3 and Dubowitz, 1989). Seventy-four patients (38 males and 36 females) were collected by our polycentric study. The mean age at the time of the first clinical evaluation was more than 13 years, the mean age at onset of the disease was 4.3 years (range: 4 months–40 years), 3.2 years for girls and 5.4 for boys.

Table 3. Mild SMA

(Kugelberg–Welander disease)

Definition	**Investigations**
An autosomal recessive disorder characterized by proximal weakness, predominantly of the legs, due to degeneration of the anterior horn cells of the spinal cord	CK: normal or moderately elevated Ultrasonography: characteristic picture of increased muscle echo plus loss of muscle bulk EMG: evidence of denervation and re-innervation
Age of onset	**Muscle biopsy**
From the second year of life through childhood and adolescence into childhood	Characteristic pattern of large group atrophy plus variable groups of normal or enlarged fibres, often uniformly type 1; or retention of normal bundle architecture with fibre type grouping, and focal small group atrophy
Presenting symptoms	
Difficulty with activities such as running, climbing steps, or jumping	
Limitation in walking ability – quality or quantity	**Genetics**
Cardinal clinical signs	Autosomal recessive; single gene for varying severities
Abnormal gait; waddling, flat-footed, wide base	
Difficulty in rising from floor (Gower's sign)	Allelic – located on chromosome 5q13.1
Proximal weakness; legs > arms	Less common dominant and X-linked forms
Hand tremor (variable)	**Management**
Tongue fasciculation (variable)	Encourage activity and ambulation
Associated features	Rehabilitation in calipers if ambulation lost
Hypermobility of joints, especially hands and feet	Vigorous treatment of respiratory infections
Course and prognosis	
Weakness usually relatively static; in some may be progressive	
Good long-term survival, depending on respiratory function	

By kind permission of Professor Dubowitz.

Here again, we have found an earlier onset in girls than boys; this interesting aspect of the disease has been reported in the literature (Hausmanowa-Petrusewicz et al., 1976; Tonali et al., 1984), and seems to be quite reliable, even if more data is necessary to confirm it (Benady, 1978; Russman et al., 1983).

Further observation

Only a small percentage of patients affected by SMA III presented a reduction of active foetal movements (8 per cent), hypotonia at birth (7 per cent), depressed spontaneous motility at birth (3 per cent) or a slight delay in motor development (16 per cent).

Triggering events are reported for eight cases: in three, disease onset was correlated with vaccination, in three others to infectious diseases and in two to trauma. It is our opinion that these are just coincidental.

Follow-up

Seventeen out of 74 patients (13 males and four females) were followed up for at least 6 years either in Pavia or at the Neurological Clinic in Padua.

Their age at the first clinical evaluation ranged from 2 to 36 years; their age at the last check-up ranged from 8 to 43 years. Fifty per cent of these 17 patients have worsened during follow-up. We have not detected worsening in another 20 per cent, probably because their clinical situation was already severe at the first work up (long-lasting disease).

Familial cases

Eight cases belonged to three kin groups. We observed variation in the age at onset and in the clinical course of the disease. Although this group is of just eight patients, it may be noted that the clinical course of the disease is more favourable in females than in males, as has already been reported by Tonali et al. (1994).

Conclusions

We have reported the findings of both a polycentric transversal study and from a longitudinal study carried out in cooperation with the Neurological Clinic at Padua. Our aim was to contribute to a better definition of SMA and its clinical progression, a problem that continues to stimulate debate (e.g. the contributions of Dubowitz in 1995 and Hausmanowa-Petrusewicz et al. in 1992).

Our data on SMA I seem to be conclusive, and almost all our patients are now dead. Longer term follow-up is, however, needed to understand the clinical progression of SMA II and III, and to identify any indices for prognosis: this will be our next goal.

References

Appelbaum, J.S., Roos, R.P., Salazar-Grueso, E.F., Buchman, A., Iannaccone, S., Glantz, R., Siddique, T. & Maselli, R. (1992): Intrafamilial heterogeneity in hereditary motor neuron disease. *Neurology* **42**, 1488–1492.

Balottin, U., Castellani, G., Fioravanti, L., Comelli, D., Ottolini, A. & Lanzi, G. (1991): Neuropsychiatric approach to a child with spinal muscular atrophy. A study of relational problems. *Minerva Pediatr.* **43**, 631–636.

Benady, S.G. (1978): Spinal muscular atrophy in childhood review of 50 cases. *Develop. Med. Child. Neurol.* **20**, 746–757.

Brzustowicz, L.M., Merette, C., Kleyn, P.W., Lehner, T., Castilla, L.H., Penchaszadeh, G.K., Das, K., Munsat, T.L., Ott, J. & Gilliam, T.C. (1993): Assessment of non allelic genetic heterogeneity of chronic (type II and III) spinal muscular atrophy. *Hum. Hered.* **43**, 380–387.

Brzustowicz, L.M., Wilhelmsen, K.C. & Gilliam, T.C. (1991): Genetic analysis of childhood-onset spinal muscular atrophy. *Adv. Neurol.* **56**, 181–187.

Byers, K.R. & Banker, Q.B. (1961): Infantile muscular atrophy. *Arch. Neurol.* **5**, 38–62.

Cerveri, I., Fanfulla, F., Zoia, M.C., Manni, R. & Tartara, A. (1993): Sleep disorders in neuromuscular diseases. *Monaldi. Arch. Chest. Dis.* **48**, 318–321.

Davies, K.E., Thomas, N.H., Daniels, R.J. & Dubowitz, V. (1991): Molecular studies of spinal muscular atrophy. *Neuromusc. Disord.* **1**, 83–85.

Davies, K. & Munsat, T. (1995): SMA Consortium, summary of meeting, 4–6 March 1994, Naarden, The Netherlands. *Neuromusc. Disord.* **5**, 333–336.

Dubowitz, V. (1964): Infantile muscular atrophy: a prospective study with particular reference to a slowly progressive variety. *Brain* **87**, 707–718.

Dubowitz, V. (1989): *A colour atlas of muscle disorders in childhood.* London: Wolfe Medical.

Dubowitz, V. (1991): Chaos in classification of the spinal muscular atrophies of childhood [editorial comments]. *Neuromusc. Disord.* **1**, 77–80.

Dubowitz, V. (1995): Chaos in the classification of SMA: a possible resolution. *Neuromusc. Disord.* **1**, 3–5.

Emery, A.E. (1991): Clinical and genetic heterogeneity in spinal muscular atrophy – the multiple allele model [letter]. *Neuromusc. Disord.* **1**, 307–308.

Emery, A.E., Davie, M.A., Holloway, S. & Skinner, R. (1976): International collaborative study of the spinal muscular atrophies. *J. Neurol. Sci.* **30**, 375–384.

Fidzianska, A., Goebel, H.H. & Warlo, I. (1990): Acute infantile spinal muscular atrophy: muscle apoptosis as a proposed pathogenetic mechanism. *Brain* **113**, 433–445.

Fischbeck, K. (1989): Reports of workshop on SMA, 19 Feb. 1989 (ENMC–AFM), p. 4.

Genneralli, M., Melchionda, S., Fattorini, C., Novelli, G. & Dallapiccola, B. (1992): Genotyping of spinal muscular atrophy families with linked DNA probes. *Clin. Genet.* **42**, 317–312.

Gordon, N. (1991): The spinal muscular atrophies. *Dev. Med. Child. Neurol.* **33**, 934–938.

Greensmith, L. & Vrabova, G. (1995): Possible strategies for treatment of SMA patients: a neurobiologist's view. *Neuromusc. Disord.* **5**, 359–369.

Grimm, T. (1989): Reports of workshop on SMA, 19 Feb. 1989 (ENMC–AFM), p. 5.

Hausmanowa-Petrusewicz, I. (1991): Spinal muscular atrophies: how many types? *Adv. Neurol.* **56**, 157–167.

Hausmanowa-Petrusewicz, I., Badurska-Modrzycka, B. & Ryniewicz, B. (1992): On chaos in classification of childhood spinal muscular atrophy [letter; comment]. *Neuromusc. Disord.* **2**, 429–430.

Hausmanowa-Petrusewicz, I., Zaremba, J., Borkowska, J. & Prot, G. (1976): Genetic investigation on chronic forms of infantile and juvenile spinal muscular atrophy. *J. Neurol.* **213**, 335–346.

Hausmanowa-Petrusewicz, I. (1993): Diagnostic methods in childhood spinal muscular atrophy. *Acta Cardiomiol.* **1**, 17–23.

Henderson, C.E., Bloch-Gallego, E., Camu, W., Gouin, A., Lemeulle, C. & Mettling, C. (1993): Motoneuron survival factors: biological roles and therapeutic potential. *Neuromusc. Disord.* **3**, 455–458.

Hoffmann, J. (1893): Ueber cronische spinale Muskelatrophie in Kindesalter auf familiarer Basis. *Dtsch. Z. Nervenheilkd* **3**, 427.

Iannacone, T.S., Browne, H.R., Samaha, G.F. & Buncher, R.C. DCN SMA Group (1993): Prospective study of spinal muscular atrophy before age 6 years. *Pediatr. Neurol.* **9**, 187–193.

Kleyn, P.W. & Gilliam, T.C. (1993): Progress toward cloning of the gene responsible for childhood spinal muscular atrophy. *Semin. Neurol.* **13**, 276–282.

Kugelberg, E. & Welander, L. (1954): Familiar neurogenetic (spinal?) muscular atrophy simulating ordinary proximal dystrophy. *Acta Psychiatr. Neurol. Scand.* **29**, 42–43.

Lanzi, G., Balottin, U., Borgatti, R. & Ottolini, A. (1993): Relational and therapeutic aspects of children with late onset of a terminal disease. *Child Nerv. Syst.* **9**, 339–342.

Lanzi, G., Besana, D., Burgio, F.R. & Lorini, R. (1977): Le amiotrofie spinali progressive: problemi nosografici. *Riv. Neurol.* **47**, 58–82.

La Spada, A.R., Roling, D.B., Harding, A.E.,Warner, C.L., Spiegel, R., Hausmanowa-Petrusewicz, I., Yee, W.C. & Fischbeck, K.H. (1992): Meiotic stability and genotype–phenotype correlation of the trinucleotide repeat in X-linked spinal and bulbar muscular atrophy. *Nat. Genet.* **2**, 301–304.

Lefebvre, S., Burgien, L., Reboullet S. *et al.* (1995): Identification and characterization of a spinal muscular atrophy determining gene. *Cell* **80**, 155–165.

Lusakowska, A., Penchaszadech, G., Badurska, B., Borkowska, J. & Hausmanowa-Petrusewicz, I. (1994): Clinical-genetic studies of infantile and juvenile proximal spinal muscular atrophy. *Neurol. Neurochir. Pol.* **28**, Suppl. 1, 91–102.

MacKenzie, A.E., Jacob, P., Surh, L. & Besner, A. (1994): Genetic heterogeneity in spinal muscular atrophy: a linkage analysis-based assessment. *Neurology* **44**, 919–924.

Manni, R., Cerveri, I., Ottolini, A., Fanfulla, F., Zoia, M.C., Lanzi, G. & Tartara, A. (1993): Sleep related breathing patterns in patients with spinal muscular atrophy. *Ital. J. Neurol. Sci.* **14**, 565–569.

Melki, J. (1991): Localization of the spinal muscular atrophy gene by reverse genetic methods. Prospect of a gene on chromosome 5. *Rev. Prat.* **21**, 1677–1679.

Merette, C., Brzustowicz, L.M., Daniels, R.J., Davies, K.E., Gilliam, T.C., Melki, J., Munnich, A., Pericak-Vancek, M.A., Siddique, T., Voosen, B. *et al.* (1994): An investigation of genetic heterogeneity and linkage disequilibrium in 161 families with spinal muscular atrophy. *Genomics* **21**, 27–33.

Munsat, T.L. & Davies, K. (1992): International SMA Consortium meeting, 26–28 June 1992, Bonn, Germany. *Neuromusc. Disord.* **2**, 423–428.

Munsat, T.L., Skerry, L., Korf, B., Pober, B., Schapira, Y., Gascon, G.G., Rajeh, A.L., Dubowitz, B., Devies, K., Brzustowicz, L.M. & Penchaszadeh, G.K. (1990): Phenotypic heterogeneity of spinal muscular atrophy mapping to chromosome 5q11. 2–13.3 (SMA 5q). *Neurology* **40**, 1831–1836.

Oppenheim, R.W. (1991): Cell death during development of the nervous system. *Ann. Rev. Neurosci.* **14**, 453–501.

Rietschel, M., Rudnik-Schoneborn, S. & Zeres, K. (1992): Clinical variability of autosomal dominant spinal muscular atrophies. *J. Neur. Sci.* **107**, 65–73.

Roy, N., Mahadevan, M.S., McLean, M. *et al.* (1995): The gene for neuronal apoptosis inhibitory protein is partially deleted in individuals with spinal muscular atrophy. *Cell.* **80**, 167–178.

Russman, S.B., Melchreit, R. & Drennan, J.C. (1983): Spinal muscular atrophy: the natural course of disease. *Muscle Nerve* **6**, 179–181.

Sarnat, H.B. (1992): *Cerebral dysgenesis: embryology and clinical expression.* Oxford: Oxford University Press.

Simard, L.R., Vanasse, M., Rochette, C., Morgan, K., Lemieux, B., Melancon, S.B. & Labuda, D. (1992): Linkage study of chronic childhood-onset spinal muscular atrophy (SMA): confirmation of close linkage to D5S39 in French-Canadian families. *Genomics* **14** 188–190.

Thomas, N.H. & Dubowitz, V. (1994): Natural history of severe SMA. *Neuromusc. Disord.* **4**, 497–502.

Tonali, T., Servidei, S., Uncini, A., Restuccia, D. & Gallucci, G. (1984): Clinical study of proximal spinal muscular atrophy. Report on 89 cases. *Ital. J. Neurol. Sci.* **5**, 423–432.

Wang, T.G., Bach, J.R., Avilla, C., Alba, A.S. & Yang, G.F. (1994): Survival of individuals with spinal muscular atrophy on ventilatory support. *Am. J. Phys. Med. Rehabil.* **73**, 207–211.

Werdnig, G. (1891): Zwei früh infantile hereditäre Fälle von progressive Muskelatrofie unter dem Bilde der Dystrofie über auf neurotischer Grundlage. *Arch. Psychiatr.* **22**, 437.

Winsor, E.I., Murphy, G., Thomson, M.W. & Reed. T.E. (1971): Genetics of chidhood spinal muscular atrophy. *J. Med. Gen.* **8**, 143.

Chapter 9

Disorders of neuromuscular transmission in childhood

Paolo Confalonieri, Carlo Antozzi, Marina Mora and Renato Mantegazza

Department of Neuromuscular Diseases, National Neurological Institute 'Carlo Besta', Via Celoria 11, 20133 Milan, Italy

Summary

Disorders of neuromuscular transmission in children include the acquired autoimmune myasthenia gravis and several myasthenic syndromes, the diagnosis of which relies upon careful clinical evaluation and sophisticated diagnostic tests. The most frequent form is acquired autoimmune myasthenia gravis in which specific autoantibodies against the acetylcholine receptor are produced, ultimately leading to the typical fluctuating muscle weakness and fatiguability. The disease is similar to that observed in adults and can be effectively treated with anticholinesterase drugs, immunosuppression, plasma exchange and thymectomy. Myasthenic syndromes include an autoimmune form (the Lambert–Eaton syndrome) and several congenital disorders. The Lambert–Eaton myasthenic syndrome has been rarely reported in children; the disease has been related to autoantibodies against the presynaptic voltage-operated calcium channel. The congenital myasthenic syndromes, non-autoimmune in nature, are usually observed within the first months or years of life. The diagnosis of these rare disorders requires a detailed morphological assessment of the neuromuscular junction and in vitro neurophysiological studies.

The neuromuscular junction (NMJ) is a chemical synapse anatomically and functionally differentiated for the transmission of signals from the motor nerve terminal to the muscle fibre. Signal transmission occurs by the release of quanta of presynaptic acetylcholine (ACh) which then binds to postsynaptic acetylcholine receptors (AChRs). Binding leads to alterations in the permeability of the postsynaptic membrane to cations, in turn leading to a muscle action potential – the first step in the muscle contraction process (Engel, 1994a). Myasthenias are acquired or congenital alterations in the neuromuscular junction which impair the normal activity of synaptic transmission and induce muscle weakness and fatiguability (increasing weakness with muscle activity). Lesions at various points on the neuromuscular junction (Fig. 1) account for the range of myasthenic conditions. The myasthenias of childhood can be more heterogeneous than those encountered in adults, and the clinician evaluating children with muscle weakness must consider not only the acquired autoimmune forms but also the heterogeneous group of congenital-genetic myasthenic syndromes. A classification of NMJ disorders in childhood is shown in Table 1.

The symptoms of these conditions, which often overlap, typically include hypotonia and cyanosis at birth, poor suckling and weak crying in the early postnatal days, and variably fluctuating weakness of the cranial, extraocular, skeletal or respiratory muscles in the ensuing years. Only by being thoroughly familiar with the clinical features, the diagnostic tests (involving morphological, immunological and neurophysiological studies) and with what is known of the pathogenetic mechanisms of these illnesses, can the physician hope to formulate an accurate prognosis and successfully manage affected children.

Table 1. Classification of childhood disorders of the neuromuscular junction

Acquired autoimmune myasthenia gravis
    Transient neonatal myasthenia gravis (TNMG)
    Juvenile myasthenia gravis (JMG)
Congenital-genetic myasthenic syndromes
Lambert–Eaton myasthenic syndrome
Penicillamine-induced myasthenia gravis
Infantile botulism

Acquired autoimmune myasthenia gravis

Myasthenia gravis (MG) is an acquired autoimmune disorder associated with functional impairment of acetylcholine receptors at the neuromuscular junction. In most patients anti-acetylcholine receptor antibodies can be detected in peripheral blood (Engel, 1994b). MG, which has an incidence estimated at between 0.5 and 3 per 100,000 in the general population (Fenichel, 1978), is the most frequent NMJ disorder in childhood. The condition is divided into two general types: transient neonatal myasthenia and juvenile myasthenia gravis.

Transient neonatal myasthenia gravis (TNM)

Transient weakness occurs in 10–15 per cent of infants born to mothers with MG (Wise & McQuillen, 1970). The symptoms arise from the presence of maternal anti-acetylcholine receptor antibodies transferred across the placenta. The clinical status of the mother at the time of pregnancy correlates poorly with the infant's risk of expressing TNMG symptoms (Elias et al., 1979). A single report describes arthrogryposis associated with severe TNMG in two infants born to the same myasthenic mother (Moutard-Codou et al., 1987). Symptoms usually appear within the first few hours of birth and last 1–4 weeks, though rarely may persist for months (Branch et al., 1978); they consist of weak suckling, diffuse muscle weakness, dysphagia, ptosis, and hypotonia. Suckling

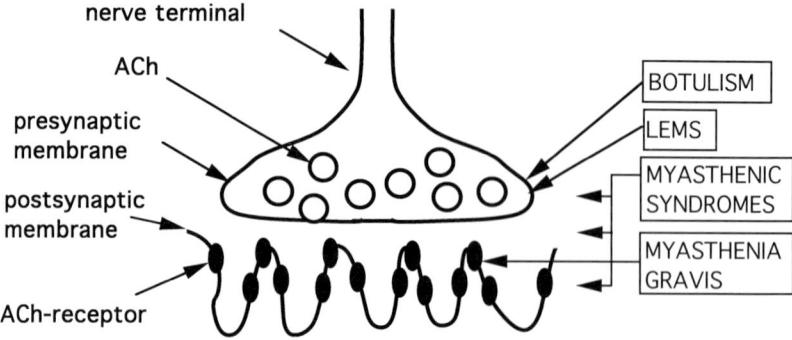

Fig. 1. Diagram of the neuromuscular junction and location of the NMJ lesion in different myasthenic conditions.

difficulties occur in 90 per cent of cases and sometimes necessitate gavage feeding. Generalized weakness and respiratory problems are present in 60–70 per cent. The administration of anticholinesterase medication produces improvement. Anti-AChR antibodies are usually detected for several days in most newborns of myasthenic mothers, and their detectability is independent from the clinical expression of the disease. Suspected or evident signs of NMJ dysfunction can be confirmed by administration of anticholinesterase agents. Very low doses (not exceeding 0.15 mg/kg subcutaneously or intramuscularly) of edrophonium chloride (Tensilon) have been recommended in such cases. Before and after Tensilon administration, it is important to check the performance of specific actions such as co-ordinated powerful sucking, head control and power on withdrawal from noxious stimuli; a clinical improvement occurs within 30–60 s of administration and lasts 4–5 min. If necessary, the condition can be confirmed by electrodiagnostic studies, using repetitive nerve stimulation rates of 2–5 Hz to elicit the typical decremental response. The risk that a child with TNMG will later develop JMG is apparently extremely low (Pirskanen, 1977; Szobor, 1989).

Juvenile myasthenia gravis (JMG)

Juvenile MG resembles the adult form with regard to clinical features and disease course (Engel, 1994b). About 10–15 per cent of all patients with acquired autoimmune MG are children. In nearly all patients with JMG, symptoms appear after the first year of age and frequently after the age of 10. In our series of 29 JMG patients, onset was between 2 and 16 years, but mean age of onset was 11.7 years and only four patients were symptomatic before the age of 10. We observed more affected girls than boys (82.7 per cent vs 17.3 per cent), as reported for adult cases. Indeed, there are no clinical or biological reasons to consider JMG as a different disease.

Abnormal weakness and fatiguability can affect all voluntary muscles, but the ocular muscles are affected initially in about 50 per cent of patients who present diplopia and ptosis of the eyelids (Engel, 1994b). Other voluntary muscles innervated by cranial nerves (facial, masticatory, lingual

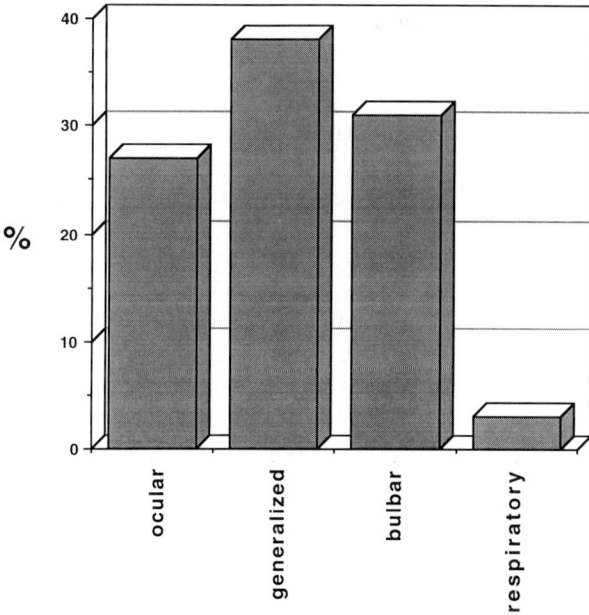

Fig. 2. Juvenile myasthenia gravis: symptoms at onset.

and pharyngeal muscles) are often involved. In our series (Fig. 2), onset was marked by ocular symptoms in only 27.5 per cent, other cranial nerve signs in 31.1 per cent, and skeletal muscle involvement in 37.9 per cent; one patient (3.5 per cent) presented respiratory insufficiency. The symptoms characteristically fluctuate daily, weekly, or over longer periods. Muscle assessment can be difficult because of poor collaboration in very young children. The frequency of associated diseases is usually high (up to 44 per cent) (Carter-Snead et al., 1980).

Table 2. Diagnosis of juvenile myasthenia gravis

Clinical history and evaluation
Clinical response to edrophonium injection
EMG with repetitive nerve stimulation
Ddetermination of serum anti-AChR antibody titre
Mediastinum CT scan/MRI

JMG is diagnosed (Table 2) on the basis of clinical examination, response to injecting anticholinesterase drugs (edrophonium chloride), electromyographic studies, and anti-AChR antibody assay in the serum. Electromyography (with repetitive nerve stimulation) is useful both in children and adults. Stimulation is most sensitive and reliable at the rate of 2–3 Hz, with maximal pathological decremental response usually obtained at the fifth evoked response. Both distal and proximal muscles are tested to increase the likelihood of detecting the typical myasthenic decrement. Difficulties may arise in very young children due to poor relaxation and movement, in which case single-fibre EMG (SFEMG) testing may be performed under sedation.

The intravenous test dose of edrophonium chloride in children weighing up to 34 kg is 0.1 ml; children weighing less receive 0.05 ml. A positive response is a decrease in muscle weakness (evaluating ptosis and/or strength of a clearly affected muscle group) appearing within 1–2 min and lasting less than 5 min.

The presence of anti-acetylcholine receptor antibodies (AChR-Ab) in sera confirms the diagnosis (Bartoccioni et al., 1986); the frequency of seronegative patients (24.2 per cent in our series) seems to be higher in children than in adult MG patients (Engel, 1994b). AChR antibody titles do not correlate with severity of disease or with treatment. When young patients with myasthenic symptoms are repeatedly seronegative, the possibility of a congenital form of myasthenia must be considered, and more complex diagnostic tests may have to be performed.

The diagnostic approach to each patient must always include the radiological evaluation of mediastinum (by contrast enhanced CT scan – MRI) to detect signs of thymic enlargement.

Treatment for JMG patients (Table 3) almost always begins with the anticholinesterase pyridostigmine bromide. This usually produces satisfactory symptom control in the early stages of the disease. The starting dose is 15–30 mg administered every 3–4 hours, then increased according to the residual clinical disability. Although experience suggests that steroid therapy is more effective than anticholinesterase therapy against extraocular muscle weakness, the risks of long-term treatment with corticosteroids must be weighed against the reported high incidence of spontaneous improvement and remission in children with ocular JMG (Dechamps et al., 1987; Rodriguez et al., 1983). Failure to achieve a satisfactory improvement (and particularly the presence of severe generalized and/or bulbar impairment) suggests the initiation of prednisone, usually at 0.5–1 mg/kg. After prednisone has produced clinical stabilization, the regimen is changed to a dose every other day, then slowly reduced to the lowest level that effectively controls symptoms.

Azathioprine and other immunosuppressants are of limited use in the treatment of JMG. Usually they are only given to patients over 10 years of age in whom the side effects of prednisone are unacceptable. As reported for adult MG, plasma exchange is extremely useful in the management of JMG crises and can be life-saving when the bulbar and respiratory muscles are severely involved (Dau et al., 1977). Limitations to the use of plasma exchange in children are mainly related to vascular access and poor collaboration. Moreover, since plasma exchange is not completely devoid of side effects, it should be considered as an emergency measure in children affected with severe generalized or fulminant MG.

Table 3. Therapy for juvenile myasthenia gravis

Pyridostigmine bromide	Every 3–4 h
	15–60 mg
Prednisone	0.5–1 mg/kg body weight/day
Azathioprine	2–3 mg/kg/day
Plasma exchange	Useful in JMG crises

The role of thymus in the pathogenesis of autoimmune myasthenia gravis is still under investigation but several findings suggest its active involvement, as demonstrated by the clinical response to thymectomy and the occurrence of thymic hyperplasia or thymoma in MG patients (Cornelio et al., 1993). Indeed, the thymus contains the cellular components required for antigen processing and presentation and likely to be involved in (and possibly initiate) the autoimmune response. Myoid cells expressing AChR are present within thymic tissue in close relationship with interdigitating cells bearing HLA class II molecules and able to function as antigen-presenting cells (Schluep et al., 1987). Moreover, hyperplastic thymuses in MG are rich in AChR-specific T cells (Melms et al., 1988).

Thymectomy is an established therapeutic procedure in adults with myasthenia gravis. The majority of retrospective reports also suggest that the procedure provides significant benefits in children. The proportion of JMG patients who improve clinically or remit is greater among those undergoing thymectomy than not (Adams et al., 1990; Sarnat et al., 1977). Twenty-four out of 29 (82.7 per cent) JMG patients from our series underwent thymectomy; of these 18 (82 per cent) had thymic hyperplasia, 14 per cent had atrophy and 4 per cent thymoma.

Figure 3 summarizes pharmacological therapy in our series of 29 JMG patients after a mean disease duration of 9.8 years. Half are satisfactorily controlled with anticholinesterase only; 12 per cent are treated with steroids only, while a further 24 per cent require steroids plus anticholinesterase. At last observation, four patients (13.8 per cent) were in true remission (considered as the absence of symptoms and signs of MG without any drug treatment for at least 1 year), while the majority (75.8 per cent) were improved, much improved or in pharmacological remission. Seven patients (24.2 per cent) had an unchanged or worsened clinical picture (shown in Fig. 4). The percentage of true remissions is similar to that (11.1 per cent) reported in a large series of Italian MG patients (Mantegazza et al., 1990).

Congenital myasthenic syndromes (CMS)

Congenital myasthenic syndromes are a heterogeneous group of disorders in which neuromuscular transmission is compromised by one or more specific non-immune mechanisms at various levels of the neuromuscular junction (Fig. 1). Prevalence is estimated at about 1–2 per 1 000 000. In Vincent et al.'s (1993) series, 16 of the 22 patients were male.

In the differential diagnosis of congenital and acquired autoimmune forms of myasthenia, note that patients with CMS are often characterized by delayed motor milestones in the first 2 years of life and sometimes by the presence of dysmorphic features at birth; furthermore, severe involvement of the trunk muscles often results in early postural scoliosis. There is no association with autoimmune

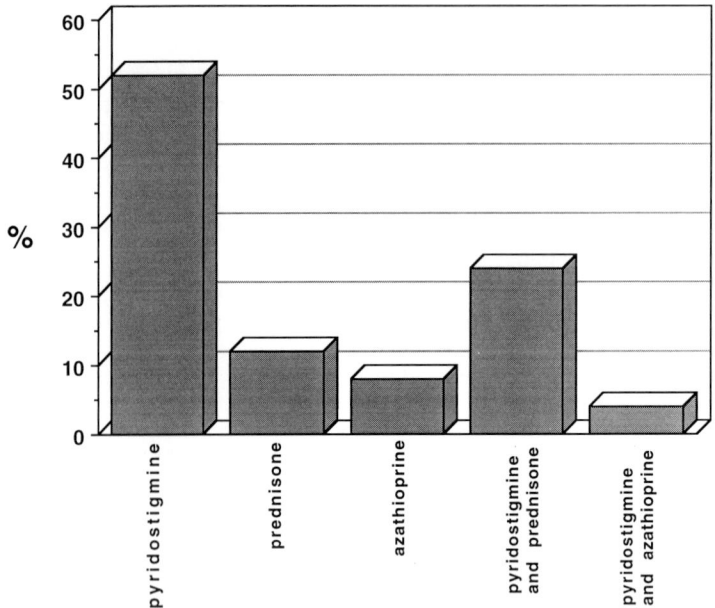

Fig. 3. Juvenile myasthenia gravis: therapy at last observation.

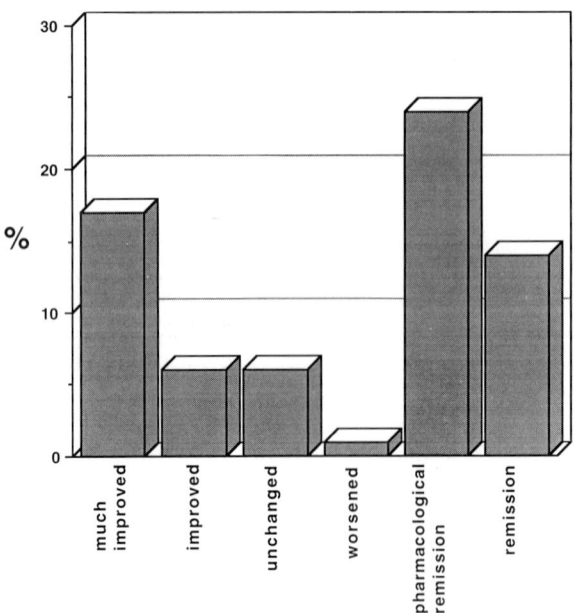

Fig. 4. Juvenile myasthenia gravis: outcome at last observation.

disease or with any particular HLA genotype. Acetylcholine receptor antibodies are absent. Maternal history, serological studies and clinical follow-up allow easy distinction between transient neonatal autoimmune myasthenia and CMS. A typical clinical history of CMS begins with ocular, bulbar, or respiratory symptoms worsened by crying or by muscle activity in infancy and childhood;

general fatiguability is often present. Symptoms usually progress in the following years (Engel, 1994c).

Differential diagnosis of the various forms of CMS is based on sophisticated morphological and electrophysiological techniques that are only rarely available to the clinician (Vincent *et al.*, 1993). Nevertheless familiarity with the more clearly defined congenital myasthenic syndromes helps to narrow diagnostic possibilities and inform prognosis and management. For this reason the diagnostic workup should be as thorough as possible (Table 4). Laboratory investigations should include electrophysiological studies (nerve conduction velocity and single and repetitive stimulation at low and high rates, before and after exercise). In vitro electrophysiological studies can identify abnormalities characteristic of specific myasthenic syndromes, but again this modality is rarely available. Muscle biopsy (preferably from an intercostal muscle) is required for electron microscope investigation of the motor end-plates and for morphological and immunochemical assays that may detect specific defects (Engel, 1994c).

Table 4. Investigation of congenital myasthenic syndromes

Clinical
    History, examination, response to AChE inhibitor
    EMG: conventional, stimulation studies, SFEGM
    Serological tests (AChR antibodies, tests for botulism)
Morphological studies
    Routine histochemical studies
    Cytochemical and immunocytochemical localizations of AChE, AChR, ACh subunits
    Eestimation of AChE-reactive end plates
    Quantitative electron microscopy and ultrastructural cytochemistry of the NMJ
Alpha-bungarotoxin binding sites on the NMJ
    In vitro electrophysiology studies
    Conventional microelectrode studies
    Noise analysis: channel kinetics
    Single-channel patch-clamp recordings

For many of the congenital myasthenic syndromes, only a single case has been reported. We provide two provisional classifications of these conditions. The first (Table 5) proposed by Engel (1994c) is based on the site of the defect. The second (Table 6) (and not yet published) was presented at the 34th European Neuromuscular Centre International Workshop (The Netherlands, June 1995) and is based on the type of inheritance. The main goal of the clinician in relation to the plethora of congenital forms of myasthenia is to distinguish them from acquired autoimmune forms. This constitutes the important first step towards rational therapy and appropriate genetic counselling. In what follows we briefly describe some of the more distinct congenital myasthenias.

Familial infantile myasthenia

First described in 1960 by Greer & Schotland, this condition is inherited in an autosomal recessive manner. Onset is usually in the neonatal period often with hypotonia and cyanosis but typically with poor suckling and weak crying. Facial weakness with fluctuating ptosis may be prominent without involvement of the extraocular muscles. Episodes of apnoea can be frequent and patients may need respiratory assistance. Differential diagnosis from transient myasthenia gravis is based on maternal history and serological investigations. Improvement usually begins spontaneously with a tendency towards remission in the following years, but some patients may complain of easy fatiguability induced by exercise. Episodic crises characterized by severe weakness, respiratory failure and death can occur (Conomy *et al.*, 1975); these may be precipitated by non-specific infections, so parents should be warned of the dangers of even trivial illnesses.

Table 5. Classification of congenital myasthenic syndromes

Presynaptic defects
Defect in ACh resynthesis or packaging ('familial infantile myasthenia')
    Paucity of synaptic vesicles and reduced release
Pre- and post-synaptic defects
    End-plate AChE deficiency
Post-synaptic defects
Kinetic abnormalities of AChR with AChR deficiency
    Classic slow-channel syndrome
    Epsilon subunit mutations with prolonged open time and low conductance of AChR channel
    AChR deficiency and short channel open time
Kinetic abnormalities of AChR without AChR deficiency
    High-conductance fast-channel syndrome
    Syndrome attributed to abnormal interaction of ACh with AChR
Partially characterized syndromes
    CMS resembling LEMS
    AChR deficiency with paucity of secondary synaptic clefts
    Other AChR deficiency
    Familial limb-girdle myasthenia
    Benign CMS with facial malformations

Anticholinesterase treatment can be effective and may be life-saving in acute crises, but response is highly variable. Non-responders should be considered for treatment with 3,4-diaminopyridine, a K^+ channel blocking agent which is able to stimulate ACh release from the nerve terminal (Shillito et al., 1993). Out of crisis, adults may show residual moderate weakness of limb or bulbar muscles.

EMG studies usually show a decremental response at 2–3 Hz stimulation in affected muscles. Electrophysiological studies in vitro suggest that the primary abnormality is a defect in acetylcholine resynthesis or mobilization, or packaging, resulting in a reduced ACh release during activity.

Table 6. Classification of myasthenic syndromes

Type I autosomal recessive
    Ia: familial infantile myasthenia
    Ib: limb girdle myasthenia
    Ic: acetylcholinesterase deficiency
    Id: acetylcholine receptor deficiency
Type II autosomal dominant
    IIIa: slow channel syndrome

End-plate acetylcholinesterase deficiency

In this autosomal recessive syndrome, the primary abnormality appears to be absence or reduction of acetylcholinesterase (AChE) at the motor endplate. AChE is the enzyme responsible for terminating the action of ACh at this site. In a review of five cases presented by Hutchinson et al. (1993), the clinical characteristics were reported as generalized weakness, present from an early age and increased by exertion, slow pupillary light responses, postural and then fixed spinal column deformity, decremental response to EMG stimulation at 2 Hz, repetitive compound muscle action potential (CMAP) following single nerve stimuli and a tendency to a slow progression with time. Typically there is no response to AChE inhibitors, so that symptom improvement following their administration may be taken to exclude this condition.

We observed (Confalonieri et al., 1994) a sporadic case of AChE deficiency in a male. Muscle weakness, muscle wasting and fatiguability had been present since the second year of life. The motor deficit worsened during the second decade but there were prolonged periods of stability. Excessive curare sensitivity was noted at age 14 when respiratory failure occurred during surgery for glaucoma. Clinical examination revealed scoliosis, ptosis of the eyelids, severe generalized muscle weakness and wasting, but only mild weakness in the masticatory muscles. Clinical and neurophysiological studies were negative in the parents and sister, while in the patient the typical repetitive CMAP following single nerve stimuli was observed. Morphological studies on external intercostal muscle showed the absence of cholinesterase activity at the neuromuscular junction, both with non-specific esterase and acetylcholinesterase (AChE) stains. Ultrastructural studies on muscle end plates revealed nerve terminals of reduced size and focal degeneration of the junctional folds. Alizarin red staining showed calcium deposits at several neuromuscular junctions. The presence of calcium deposits, previously reported in one of six patients with slow channel syndrome (Engel, 1994c), may play a pathogenetic role in focal degeneration at the junctional folds.

Congenital acetylcholine receptor deficiency

Several familial and a number of sporadic cases of congenital acetylcholine receptor deficiency have been reported (Engel, 1994c). The onset may occur at birth or during childhood, with involvement of the extraocular muscles (bilateral ptosis and ophthalmoplegia). Diminished foetal movement and arthrogryposis have been reported.

EMG reveals a decremental response to stimulation at 2–3 Hz. The main abnormality is reduction in the number of AChRs as determined by α-bungarotoxin binding, associated with abnormal neuromuscular junction morphology. The course is generally benign and anticholinesterase drugs are able to improve the signs and symptoms.

Slow channel syndrome

This disorder is transmitted in an autosomal dominant mode with complete penetrance and variable clinical expression. Sporadic cases are known. The condition is characterized clinically by the typical involvement (with wasting) of the cervical and scapular muscles and finger extensors. Onset of symptoms is variable, but the condition develops more often in adolescence or adulthood than any other myasthenic syndrome. Clinical progression is highly variable with periods of partial remission or stability. As in acetylcholine receptor deficiency, a typical repetitive compound end-plate action potential is elicited in response to single nerve stimuli. Patients with this disease are made worse by anti-AChE preparations and no useful drug therapy is currently available. Electrophysiological studies indicate that a prolonged open time of the ion channel traversing the acetylcholine receptor (Fig. 1) is the defect responsible for the disease (Engel et al., 1982).

Lambert–Eaton myasthenic syndrome

The Lambert–Eaton myasthenic syndrome (LEMS) is an acquired autoimmune disease in which autoantibodies deplete the voltage-sensitive calcium channels of the motor nerve terminal by antigenic modulation (Sher et al., 1989; Leys et al., 1989; Lennon & Lambert, 1989; Lang et al., 1993) (Fig. 1). In two-thirds of male patients LEMS is a paraneoplastic syndrome, the majority of tumours being small-cell carcinoma of the lung, the cells of which express voltage-sensitive calcium channels (Comola et al., 1993). The non-neoplastic form, affecting the remaining third of patients, is often associated with other autoimmune diseases. The age of onset for this form varies and may be in the first decade (Engel, 1994c). Symptoms are weakness and fatiguability typically involving trunk and limb muscles. Ocular symptoms are usually mild and transient. Proximal lower limb muscles are severely involved in most patients which frequently show autonomic nervous system abnormalities such as reduced salivation, lachrymation and sweating; orthostatic hypotension, impaired pupillary reflexes and impotence have been reported. Diagnosis is based on clinical features and electrophysiological findings. An incremental response to repetitive nerve stimulation at rates above 10 Hz is found – a response pattern opposite to that seen in MG patients. An immunoprecipitation assay recently developed to detect antibodies to P-type voltage-gated calcium channels detected these antibodies in 56 of 66 patients in one series of LEMS patients, both with and without cancer. This assay is therefore useful for diagnosing the condition (Motomura et al., 1995). 3,4-Diaminopyridine is effective in relieving both the motor and autonomic symptoms of LEMS; the most used treatment for non-neoplastic LEMS is prednisone every other day associated with 1.5–2 mg/kg/day of azathioprine. Plasmapheresis has been effective in some cases (Streib & Rothner, 1981; Engel, 1994c).

Penicillamine–induced myasthenia gravis

D-Penicillamine is used in the treatment of rheumatoid arthritis, Wilson's disease, and cystinuria. After taking this drug for several months, tolerance to self-AChR can be reversibly broken in susceptible individuals, with the consequent induction of myasthenia gravis. This form of MG is characterized by mild weakness, frequently restricted to ocular muscles and the presence of anti-AChR antibodies in serum. Symptoms usually disappear slowly after the drug is discontinued (Bucknall et al., 1975), and treatment with anticholinesterase drugs is often all that is required during this period.

Infantile botulism

The anaerobic bacterium *Clostridium botulinum* produces a toxin which blocks the release of ACh from motor nerve terminals (Fig. 1), causing severe long-lasting muscle paralysis, otherwise known as botulism. Infantile botulism occurs following chronic absorption of small quantities of the toxin (Johnson et al., 1979) or when the bacterium grows in the gastrointestinal tract. Onset is usually at about 4 months of age, with constipation, lethargy, poor suckling and weak crying as the main symptoms. On examination, the limb and oropharyngeal muscles are weak. The condition may be severe enough to require respiratory support and is a known cause of sudden death in infants. EMG studies show a typical incremental response greater than 20 per cent at stimulation rates of 20 to 50 Hz (Cornblath et al., 1983). Treatment consists of bivalent or trivalent antitoxin, but is primarily supportive, with respiratory assistance when necessary; guanidine or 4-aminopyridine may improve symptoms but do not shorten disease.

References

Adams, C., Theodorescu, D., Murphy, E.G. & Shandling, B. (1990): Thymectomy in juvenile myasthenia gravis. *J. Child. Neurol.* **5**, 216.

Bartoccioni, E., Evoli, A., Casali, C., Scoppetta, C., Tonali, P. & Provenzano, C. (1986): Neonatal myasthenia gravis: clinical and immunological study of seven mothers and their newborn infants. *J. Neuroimmunol.* **12**, 55–161.

Branch, C.E., Swift, T.R. & Dyken, P.R. (1978): Prolonged neonatal myasthenia gravis: electrophysiological studies. *Ann. Neurol.* **3**, 416–418.

Bucknall, R.C., Dixon, A.J., Glick, E.N., Woodland, J. & Zutshi, D.W. (1975): Myasthenia gravis associated with penicillamine treatment for rheumatoid arthritis. *Br. Med. J.* **i**, 600–602.

Carter-Snead, O., Benton, J.W., Dwyer, D., Morley, B., Kemp, G.E., Bradley, R.J. & Oh, S.J. (1980): Juvenile myasthenia gravis. *Neurology* **30**, 732–739.

Comola, M., Nemni, R., Sher, E., Quattrini, A., Faravelli, A., Corbo, M., Clementi, F. & Canal, N. (1993): Lambert–Eaton myasthenic syndrome and polyneuropathy in a patient with epidermoid carcinoma of the lung. *Eur. Neurol.* **33**, 121–125.

Confalonieri, P., Mora, M., Morandi, L., Ciano, C., Mantegazza, R., Antozzi, C., Zuffi, M., Blasevich, F., Di Blasi, C. & Cornelio, F. (1994): Congenital myasthenic syndrome with acetylcholinesterase deficiency and calcium deposits at neuromuscular junctions. *Neuromusc. Disord.* **4,** S27.

Conomy, J.P., Levinsohn, M. & Fanaroff, A. (1975): Familial infantile myasthenia gravis: a cause of sudden death in young chidren. *J. Pediatr.* **87,** 428–429.

Cornblath, D.R., Stadky, J.T. & Summer, A.J. (1983): Clinical electrophysiology of infantile botulism. *Muscle Nerve* **6,** 448–452.

Cornelio, F., Antozzi, C., Mantegazza, R., Confalonieri, P., Berta, E., Peluchetti, D., Sghirlanzoni, A. & Fiaccino, F. (1993): Immunosuppressive treatments. Their efficacy on myasthenia gravis patients' outcome and on the natural course of the disease. *Ann. N.Y. Acad. Sci.* **681,** 594–602.

Dau, P.C., Lindstrom, J.M., Cassel, C.K., Denys, E.H., Shev, E.E. & Spittler, E.L. (1977): Plasmapheresis and immunosuppressive drug therapy in myasthenia gravis. *N. Engl. J. Med.* **297,** 1134–1140.

Dechamps, H., Bataille, J., Estournet, B. & Barois, A. (1987): La myasthenie de l'enfant: évolution à long terme. *Ann. Med. Interne.* **138,** 615.

Elias, S.B., Butler, I. & Appen, S.H. (1979): Neonatal myasthenia gravis in the infant of a myasthenic mother in remission. *Ann. Neurol.* **6,** 72.

Engel, A.G., Lambert, E.H., Mulder, D.M., Torres, C.F., Sahashi, K., Bertorini, T.O. & Whitaker, J.N. (1982): Newly recognized congenital myasthenic syndrome attributed to a prolonged open time of the acetylcholine-induced ion channel. *Ann. Neurol.* **11,** 553–569.

Engel, A.G. (1994a): The neuromuscular junction. In: *Myology*, eds. A.G. Engel & C.Franzini-Armstrong, pp. 261–302. New York: McGraw-Hill.

Engel, A.G. (1994b): Acquired autoimmune myasthenia gravis. In: *Myology*, eds. A.G. Engel & C. Franzini-Armstrong, pp. 1769–1797. New York: McGraw-Hill.

Engel, A.G. (1994c): Myasthenic syndromes. In: *Myology*, eds. A.G. Engel & C. Franzini-Armstrong, pp. 1798–1835. New York: McGraw-Hill.

Fenichel, G.M. (1978): Clinical syndromes of myasthenias in infancy and chidhood. *Arch. Neurol.* **35,** 97–103.

Greer, M. & Schotland, M. (1960): Myasthenia gravis in the newborn. *Pediatrics* **26,** 101–108.

Hutchinson, D.O., Engel, A.G., Walls, T.J., Nakano, S., Camp, S., Taylor, P., Harper, C.M. & Brengman, J.M. (1993): The spectrum of congenital end-plate acetylcholinesterase deficiency. *Ann. N. Y. Acad. Sci.* **681,** 469–486.

Johnson, R.O., Clay, S.A. & Aaron, S.S. (1979): Diagnosis and management of infantile botulism. *Am. J. Dis. Child.* **133,** 586–593.

Lang, B., Johnston, I., Leys, K., Elrington, G., Marqueze, B., Leveque, C., Martin-Moutot, N., Seagar, M., Hoshino, T., Takahashi, M., Sugimori, M., Cherksey, B.D., Linas, R. & Newsom-Davis, J. (1993): Autoantibody specificities in Lambert–Eaton myasthenic syndrome. *Ann. N. Y. Acad. Sci.* **681,** 382–393.

Lennon, V.A. & Lambert, E.H. (1989): Autoantibodies bind solubilized calcium channel-w-conotoxin complexes from small cell lung carcinoma: a diagnostic aid for Lambert–Eaton myasthenic syndrome. *Mayo Clin. Proc.* **64,** 1498–1504.

Leys, K., Lag, B., Vincent, A. & Newsom-Davies, J. (1989): Calcium channel autoantibodies in Lambert–Eaton myasthenic syndrome. *Lancet* **ii,** 1107.

Mantegazza, R., Beghi, E., Pareyson, D., Antozzi, C., Peluchetti, D., Sghirlanzoni, A., Cosi, V., Lombardi, M., Piccolo, G., Tonali, P., Evoli, A., Ricci, E., Batocchi, A.P., Angelini, C., Micaglio, G.F., Marconi, G., Taiuti, R., Bergamini, L., Durelli, L. & Cornelio, F. (1990): A multicenter follow-up study of 1152 patients with myasthenia gravis in Italy. *J. Neurol.* **237,** 339–344.

Melms, A., Schalke, B.C.G., Kirchner, T., Muller-Hermelink, H.K., Albert, E. & Wekerle, H. (1988): Thymus in myasthenia gravis. *J. Clin. Invest.* **81,** 902–908.

Motomura, M., Johnston, I., Lang, B., Vincent, A. & Newsom-Davis J. (1995): An improved diagnostic assay for Lambert–Eaton myasthenic syndrome. *J. Neurol. Neurosurg. Psychiatry* **58,** 85–87.

Moutard-Codou, M.L., Delleur, M.M., Dulac, O. *et al.* (1987): Myasthénie néonatale sévère avec arthrogripose. *Presse Med.* **16,** 615.

Pirskanen, R. (1977): Genetic aspect in myasthenia gravis. A family study of 264 Finnish patients. *Acta Neurol. Scand.* **56,** 365.

Rodriguez, M., Gomez, M., Howard, F.M. & Taylor, W.F. (1983): Myasthenia gravis in children: long term follow-up. *Ann. Neurol.* **13,** 504.

Sarnat, H.B., McGarry, J.D. & Lewis, J.E. (1977): Effective treatment of infantile myasthenia gravis by combined prednisone and thymectomy. *Neurology* **27**, 550.

Schluep, M., Willcox, N., Vincent, A., Dhoot, G.K. & Newsom-Davis, J. (1987): Acetylcholine receptors in human thymic myoid cells in situ: an immunohistological study. *Ann. Neurol.* **22**, 212–222.

Sher, E., Gotti, C., Canal, N., Piccolo, G., Evoli, A. & Clementi, F. (1989): Specificity of calcium channel autoantibodies in Lambert–Eaton myasthenic syndrome. *Lancet* **ii**, 640–643.

Shillito, P., Vincent, A. & Newsom-Davis, J. (1993): Congenital myasthenic syndromes. *Neuromusc. Disord.* **3**, 183–190.

Streib, E.W. & Rothner, A.D. (1981): Eaton–Lambert myasthenic syndrome: long-term treatment of three patients with prednisone. *Ann. Neurol.* **10**, 488.

Szobor, A. (1989): Myasthenia gravis: familial occurrence. A study of 1100 myasthenia gravis patients. *Acta Med. Hung.* **46**, 13–21.

Vincent, A., Newsom-Davies, J., Wray, D., Shillito, P., Harrison, J., Betty, M., Beeson, D., Mills, K., Palace, J., Molenaar, P. & Murray, N. (1993): Clinical and experimental observation in patients with congenital myasthenic syndromes. *Ann. N.Y. Acad. Sci.* **61**, 451–460.

Wise, G.A. & McQuillen, M.P. (1970): Transient neonatal myasthenia. *Arch. Neurol.* **22**, 556.

Chapter 10

Current concepts review on the orthopaedic treatment of muscular diseases in childhood

Francesco Motta and Sergio Monforte

Department of Paediatric Orthopaedics, Bassini Hospital,
Cinisello Balsamo, Milan, Italy

Summary

The authors present the current knowledge on the orthopaedic treatment of the most common muscular diseases in childhood. Explaining the orthopaedic and surgical approaches to this deformities they underline the relatively limited goals of surgery.

The muscular dystrophies constitute a group of chronic muscle diseases whose main characteristic is degeneration of skeletal muscle. The primary disease process is degeneration of the muscle cell; the condition is non-inflammatory and has no associated central nervous system abnormality. The disease is transmitted genetically although a mutation may result in spontaneous occurrence.

The different types of dystrophy are characterized by age of onset, groups of muscles first affected, genetic transmission, and parts of the body with progressive weakness (Duchenne, 1868).

Common muscular dystrophies with specific orthopaedic deformities include sex-linked conditions, including Duchenne's muscular dystrophy (DMD), Becker's muscular dystrophy (BMD) and Emery–Dreifuss dystrophy; those with recessive transmission, such as congenital dystrophy and limb-girdle muscular dystrophy; and those with dominant transmission, such as facioscapulohumeral muscular dystrophy, scapuloperoneal dystrophy, oculopharyngeal dystrophy, and distal dystrophy (Thomas et al., 1986).

After the family history has been obtained and a physical examination has been performed, tests are needed to confirm the presence and to specify the type of neuromuscular disease.

Traditionally, these diagnostic studies have included measurement of levels of muscle enzymes (creatinine phosphokinase and aldolase) (Munsat et al., 1969), electrophysiological studies (EMG and nerve conduction), and muscle and nerve biopsies.

Each symptom in the patient's history must be pursued to determine onset of the disease, duration, exacerbating or relieving factors, and response to any treatment.

Orthopaedic management

The common orthopaedic problems in children with muscular dystrophy include contractures, postural foot deformities, dislocation of the hip, scoliosis and fractures (Armstrong et al.,1971; Brooke et al., 1989; McComb et al., 1979).

Contractures: upper extremities

Contractures of the upper extremities in association with decreased muscle function invariably occur in patients with DMD; the contractures worsen considerably during the second decade of life (Shapiro et al., 1993).

Adduction contractures of the shoulder and flexion contractures of the elbow are not a functional problem in themselves, as muscle weakness renders the patient unable to abduct the arm above the level of the shoulder or to extend the elbow against gravity.

The contractures do not preclude functioning for patients who must use a wheelchair, despite the diminished levels of strength. Patients who also have DMD also present pronation contractures of the forearm and flexion contracture of the elbow, wrist and fingers.

In children who have limb-girdle dystrophy, the disease may occur in the first to fourth decades of life; the later the onset, the more rapid the progression. Upper extremity weakness may involve the trapezius, the serratus anterior, the rhomboids, the latissimus dorsi, and the pectoralis major. Some weakness may develop in the prime movers of the fingers and wrist as well.

Facioscapulohumeral muscular dystrophy is characterized by weakness of the facial and shoulder-girdle muscle. Onset of the disease may occur in early childhood or in adulthood (15–35 years). In the infantile form, the disease runs a rapid, progressive course, confining most children to a wheelchair by the age of 8 to 9 years.

The greatest functional impairments are the inability to abduct and flex the arms at the glenohumeral joints and winging of the scapula, both caused by the progressive weakness of the muscles that fix the scapula to the thoracic wall, while the muscles that abduct the glenohumeral joint remain strong.

Orthopaedic management of orthopaedic deformities of upper extremities include daily, passive range of motion exercises, useful in minimizing contractures. When passive dorsiflexion of the wrist is limited to neutral, we recommend that the patient should wear orthoses at night.

A surgical approach will be only for selected patients with specific functional problems, for the use of a computer or an electrical wheelchair (Shapiro et al., 1993). In facioscapulohumeral dystrophy, particularly in the infantile form, we use surgical stabilization of the scapulothoracic region with strut grafts or with plates and screws as described by Letournel et al. (1990) to improve abduction of the shoulder.

Contractures: lower extremities

Contractures and progressive weakness of the lower extremities render walking increasingly difficult in patients with muscular dystrophy. The condition is generally not detected at birth, unlike congenital muscular dystrophy.

Early developmental milestones such as as rolling, sitting and standing are reached within the normal age limits. However, once a child stands and walks, the condition can be easily detected. Weakness, beginning in the proximal muscle groups and descending symmetrically in both lower extremities, is reflected by changes in the child's posture and gait.

In the early stage of ambulation, excessive plantar flexion may be seen during swing with a compensatory increase in hip flexion to clear the foot. Initial contact is with the foot flat to minimize the flexion torque at the hip and knee (Hsu, 1993). In the transitional stage of ambulation, increasing muscle weakness results in compensatory changes in body alignment.

In the frontal plane, the base of support is widened with an increase in lateral arm swing and trunk lean to compensate for gluteus medius weakness. Poor hip extensor strength cannot resist normal hip flexion demands at loading response (Hsu, 1993). In the late stage of ambulation, muscle weakness has progressed to the point when the child falls frequently. The base of support is widened further and step length is decreased. An increase in anterior pelvic tilt causes the child to increase his lordosis and move his arms further behind the hip joint. Toe walking is noted. Floor contact is forefoot first, which stabilizes the knee as the tibia thrusts backward; thus contact and the resulting knee flexion is avoided. In Duchenne's muscular dystrophy the average patient is unable to walk effectively by a time varying from 8 to 14 years in the absence of treatment.

When these patients stop walking, they become more susceptible to the development of scoliosis. Contractures are inevitable in these patients, but controlling their severity enhances the quality of life.

Toe walking, caused by contractures of the Achilles tendon, can sometimes be detected in patients as young as 3 years of age, and it responds to stretching therapy or to serial stretching walking plaster casts. Tendon lengthening in young ambulatory patients is discouraged because of the resulting weakness.

For the ambulatory patient, a night-time ankle foot orthosis helps to eliminate the typical equinus posturing of the foot during sleep, and muscle stretching therapy delays progression of contractures.

Despite aggressive therapy, the ability to walk becomes threatened between the ages of 8 and 12 years (transitional phase) from muscle weakness; contractures of the hip flexors, hamstring muscles, and iliotibial tract, and equinovarus deformities of the feet occur also.

If walking is severely compromised, surgery for these contractures, with immediate long leg bracing, reportedly extends the ability to walk by 1 to 5 years (Bowker et al., 1978; Curtis et al., 1970; Vignos et al., 1963).

Long leg orthoses are mandatory after surgical release of contractures and this fact must be clearly understood by the family. Common procedures used to treat contractures of the lower extremities in children with muscular dystrophy include Yount fasciotomy of the iliotibial tract, Ober release of the iliotibial band, distal release of hamstring muscles, transfer of the posterior tibialis tendon to the dorsum of the foot, or percutaneous lengthening of the Achilles tendon and open lengthening of the Achilles tendon (Shapiro et al., 1993).

Most surgery is performed bilaterally in one operative procedure and lightweight long leg casts are applied with the knees in extension and with the feet neutral. Standing is begun the day after surgery, and, if tolerated, a rapid return to walking is encouraged (Canale, 1995). In most patients, orthopaedic procedures are frequently not needed until after childhood.

Contractures of the foot and overpull of the posterior tibialis muscle may be effectively treated with a minimum ambulatory approach (Achilles tendon lengthening and tendon transfer) with good long-term results (Canale, 1995).

In limb-girdle dystrophy, lower extremity weakness may involve the gluteus maximus, the iliopsoas and the quadriceps but surgery is seldom required. Although release of contractures usually allows another 2–3 years of ambulation, by the age of 12–13 years most children with DMD can no longer walk and spinal deformity becomes the primary problem (Canale, 1995).

The orthopaedic treatment of Becker's muscular dystrophy and Emery–Dreyfuss muscular dystrophy depends on the severity of the disease (Bowen, 1993; Shapiro, 1982, 1991).

Scoliosis

During walking age, spinal lordosis develops to compensate for weakness of the trunk and pelvic muscles.

By the time the child must use a wheelchair, a functional kyphosis typically develops (Bowen, 1993). Cambridge & Drennar (1987) reported that scoliosis developed in 95 per cent of their patients after loss of ambulation.

Early scoliosis develops in 25 per cent of patients while they are still able to walk (Brooke et al., 1989; Lord et al., 1990). The scoliosis is usually a long C-shaped collapsing curve that progresses steadily until a severe deformity results; it is generally centred in the lower thoracic curve or lumbar region and almost always involves the pelvis, leading to severe pelvic obliquity and difficulties in sitting (Smith et al., 1989; Shapiro et al., 1992).

Scoliosis and weakness of the thoracic muscle increase the deterioration of pulmonary function when the children are in their second decade of life. An essential linear decrease in pulmonary status occurs over time (Smith et al., 1989; Kurtz et al., 1983).

Various spinal orthoses and wheelchair adaptations have been used to control the scoliosis, but none have been totally successful and, at best, they only delayed the progression of curvature (Bowen, 1993). When the curve is still flexible and reaches about 40°, a posterior spinal fusion (Luque rod or unit rod system) from the upper thoracic area to the sacrum should be performed, if warranted by the general condition of the patient.

Given the natural history of the condition, delaying surgery until the curve reaches 40° to 50° has no advantage and may make surgery more complicated because of the decrease in cardiac and pulmonary function that progresses during the delay (Canale, 1995). After surgery, the patient should be mobilized rapidly to retain muscle strength and reduce systemic problems (Bowen, 1993).

Hip dislocation

Dislocated hips can occur at birth or develop later in children with congenital myopathies. They are usually easily reducible in early infancy, but require prolonged treatment to achieve stability. The Pavlik harness is excellent for maintaining reduction in newborns and young infants.

It is important not to allow the hip to remain persistently posteriorly dislocated in the Pavlik harness because this creates a severe treatment complication. An older child who has developed contracture of the hip or whose hip does not easily reduce initially is treated in skin traction until the femoral head approaches the area of acetabulum.

With the patient under general anaesthesia, the hip is gently reduced and a cast is applied to maintain stability. Cast treatment may be necessary for as long as 5 months. Hip dysplasia after treatment for dislocation or from hypotonia and joint laxity usually responds to abduction bracing.

After ambulation is achieved, an abduction brace is helpful, but most children have difficulty walking with the brace. If dysplasia persists despite brace therapy in an ambulating child, a varus femoral osteotomy or a pelvic osteotomy will be helpful. Muscle weakness predisposes the patient with muscular dystrophy to falls, and relative inactivity results in osteopenic bone (Bowen, 1993).

Fractures

Fractures of the long bones are a common problem that results from immobilization. Nondisplaced fractures of the femur and tibia are treated in lightweight long leg casts or splints. Weight bearing is encouraged, but bed rest and traction are contra-indicated.

Displaced fractures of the lower limbs require prompt surgical stabilization; a lightweight orthosis may be applied to the leg over the area of internal fixation, and ambulation may begin (Bowen, 1993).

Conclusions

Over the last decade there has been improved clinical, genetic, and molecular definition of inherited muscular disorders of childhood. This has allowed for a better understanding of the natural history of these disorders and, in particular, of the associated orthopaedic deformities and the results of orthopaedic treatment.

Although the possibility of a cure lies in the realm of gene therapy, informed orthopaedic management is essential to align and support the weakened musculoskeletal system (Shapiro, 1993).

References

Armstrong, R.M. *et al.* (1971): Central core disease with congenital hip dislocation in two families. *Neurology* **21**, 369.

Bowen, J.R. (1993): *Muscle and nerve disorders in children*, ed. M. Chapman. Philadelphia: Lippincott & Co./American Academy of Orthopaedic Surgeons.

Bowker, J.H. *et al.* (1978): Factors determining success in reambulation of the child with progressive muscular dystrophy. *Orthop. Clin. North Am.* **9**, 431.

Brooke, M.H. *et al.* (1989): Duchenne muscular dystrophy: patterns of clinical progression and effects of supportive therapy. *Neurology* **39**, 475–481.

Canale, S.T. (1995): *Operative pediatric orthopaedics*, 2nd ed. St. Louis: Mosby.

Cambridge, W. & Drennar, J.C. (1987): Scoliosis associated with Duchenne muscular dystrophy. *J. Pediatr. Orthop.* **7**, 436–440.

Curtis, B.H. *et al.* (1970): Orthopaedic management of muscular dystrophy and related disorders. *Instructional Course Lectures* vol. 19, p. 78. Washington DC: American Academy of Orthopaedic Surgeons.

Duchenne, G.B. (1868): Recherches sur la paralysie pseudohypertrophique ou paralysie myosclérotique. *Arch. Gen. Med.* **11**, 5.

Hsu, J.D. (1993): Gait posture in the Duchenne muscular dystrophy child. *Clin. Orthop.* **288**, 122–125.

Kurtz, L.T. *et al.* (1983): Correlation of scoliosis and pulmonary function in Duchenne muscular dystrophy. *J. Pediatr. Orthop.* **3**, 347–353.

Letournel, E. *et al.* (1990): Scapulothoracic arthrodesis for patients who have facioscapulohumeral muscular dystrophy. *J. Bone Joint Surg. [Am]* **72A**, 78–84.

Lord, J. *et al.* (1990): Scoliosis associated with Duchenne muscular dystrophy. *Arch. Phys. Med. Rehabil.* **71**, 13–17.

McComb, R.D *et al.* (1979): Fatal neonatal nemaline myopathy with multiple congenital anomalies. *J. Pediatr.* **94**, 47.

Munsat, T.L. *et al.* (1969): Centronuclear ('myotubular') myopathy. *Arch. Neurol.* **20**, 120.

Shapiro, F. *et al.* (1982): Current concepts review. Orthopaedic management of childhood neuromuscular disease, part III: diseases of muscle. *J. Bone Joint Surg. [Am]* **64A**, 1102–1107.

Shapiro, F. *et al.* (1991): Orthopedic deformities in Emery–Dreifuss muscular dystrophy. *J. Pediatr. Orthop.* **11**, 336.

Shapiro, F. *et al.* (1992): Spinal fusion in Duchenne muscular dystrophy: a multidisciplinary approach. *Muscle Nerve* **15**, 604–614.

Shapiro, F. *et al.* (1993): Current concepts review. The diagnosis and orthopaedic treatment of inherited muscular diseases of childhood. *J. Bone Joint Surg. [Am]* **75A**, 439–454.

Smith, A.D. *et al.* (1989): Progression of scoliosis in Duchenne muscular dystrophy. *J. Bone Joint Surg. [Am]* **71A**, 1066–1074.

Thomas, N.S. *et al.* (1986): Localization of the gene for Emery–Dreifuss muscular dystrophy to the distal long arm of the X chromosome. *J. Med. Genet.* **23**, 596.

Vignos, P.J. *et al.* (1963): Management of progressive muscular dystrophy in childhood. *JAMA* **184**, 89.

Chapter 11

Therapy of scoliosis in neuromuscular pathology

André J. Kaelin

Paediatric Orthopaedics Unit, Children's Hospital, 30 boulevard de la Cluse, 1211 Geneva, Switzerland

Summary

Neuromuscular diseases are very often associated with spinal deformities and imbalance. Growing spines are particularly subject to incurvation in the frontal and sagittal plane. Each neuromuscular disease has an individual prevalence of spinal deformities and risk of progression.

Treatment aims to preserve function by detecting early curves, preventing joint contractures, and maintaining the highest level of activity (ambulation, transfer, sitting position). Physical therapy and orthoses are effective adjuvant therapies in young patients and the only treatment for small scoliotic or kyphotic curves with low risk of progression. Recent technical improvements in spinal instrumentation, anaesthesiology and reanimation allow us to perform surgical correction and instrumentation of spinal deformities caused by neuromuscular diseases.

In this paper we describe the cause of neuromuscular spinal deformities, their prevalence and the surgical indications and techniques.

The spine is a flexible structure consisting of vertebrae, joints and disks supported and balanced by strong muscular groups. In the growing spine, imbalance can influence intervertebral relationships and bone shape. Neuromuscular diseases perturb muscle strength and proprioception which are mandatory for normal spinal growth. Lonstein & Renshaw (1987) stated that spinal stability is directly proportional to the condition of its end support and inversely proportional to both spinal flexibility and to the square of the spinal-column length. According to those rules, the vertebral column is specially at risk in children and adolescents with neuromuscular diseases.

Muscle functions in neuromuscular diseases are perturbed by lack of strength and flexibility, shortening, high tonus and spasticity, by the time contractures occur. Thus, as soon as the ability to balance the growing spine is impaired, this risk of developing spinal deformity appears.

Many authors (Brown & Swank, 1985; Cambridge & Drennan, 1987; Oda *et al.*, 1993; Shapiro & Specht, 1993a, 1993b; Stagnara, 1985) describe this phenomenon, emphasizing the spine's flexibility and its remaining growth, factors that are particularly important in neuromuscular scoliosis because the deformities develop at a younger age than in idiopathic scoliosis. Pelvic stability and pelvic obliquity are present mainly in patients who have lost their ability to walk and are confined to wheelchairs. The pelvis must be considered as a vertebral body in itself; its position is altered by hip joint contractures and dislocations. Balance problems while sitting are mainly due to hip contractures, then to scoliosis or kyphosis (Smith & Emans, 1992). All forms of treatment must take into account hip and pelvic imbalances.

The usual pattern of scoliosis progression cannot be applied, because neuromuscular spinal deformities continue beyond skeletal maturity, and neurological or muscular problems may also progress.

Causes of neuromuscular spinal deformities

The causes of neuromuscular scoliosis are numerous. The types of lesions and the main diagnoses are the following:

Upper motoneurone:

    Cerebral palsy (Kalen et al., 1992; Rinsky, 1990)
    Friedreich's ataxia (Labelle et al., 1986; Shapiro & Specht, 1993b)
    Brain tumour, trauma and infection
    Rett syndrome (Lindström et al., 1987)
    Familial dysautonomia or Ryley-Day syndrome

Lower motoneurone:

    Poliomyelitis (Eberle, 1988)
    Spinal muscular atrophy (Oda et al., 1993; Shapiro & Specht, 1993b)
    Paraplegia (Dearlof et al., 1990)
    Syringomyelia
    Diastematomyelia

Peripheral nerve lesions:

    Charcot–Marie–Tooth (Daher et al., 1986; Shapiro & Specht, 1993b)
    Dejerine–Sottas (Shapiro & Specht, 1993b)

Muscular lesions:

    Duchenne's muscular dystrophy (Cambridge & Drennan, 1987; Oda et al., 1993; Shapiro & Specht, 1993a; Smith et al., 1989)
    Becker's muscular dystrophy (Shapiro & Specht, 1993a)
    Congenital muscular dystrophy (Shapiro & Specht, 1993a)
    Fascioscapular dystrophy (Shapiro & Specht, 1993a)
    Ossifying myositis

Other lesions:

    Arthrogryposis (Daher et al., 1986)
    Neurofibromatosis
    Myelomeningocele.

It is not possible to describe all types of scoliosis characteristics for every syndrome. Neuromuscular curves have in common the following characteristics:

    Early onset
    Long C-curves which can include the pelvis (Fig. 1)
    Rapid progression which continues after skeletal maturity
    Pelvic obliquity
    Compromised functional abilities
    Cardiac and/or pulmonary insufficiencies.

Chapter 11   Therapy of scoliosis in neuromuscular pathology

The prevalence of spinal deformities varies depending on the neuromuscular disorders, as stated by Lonstein & Renshaw (1987):

Neuromuscular disorder	% with spinal deformity
Cerebral palsy	25
Myelomeningocele	60
Infantile quadriplegia	100
Pre-adolescent quadriplegia	90
Duchenne's muscular dystrophy	95
Spinal muscular atrophy	100
Friedreich's ataxia	95
Rett syndrome	45

Types of spinal deformity

Because of their specificity we will describe five different types of spinal deformities and their ways of progression.

1. *Duchenne's muscular dystrophy* patients develop scoliosis at a very high rate (Cambridge & Drennan, 1987; Galasko et al., 1987; Lonstein & Renshaw, 1987; Smith et al., 1989; Suzuki et al., 1993). In 75 per cent of cases incurvation of the spine appears after the loss of walking ability and in 25 per cent before. The side of the long C-shaped scoliosis depends on the side of the iliotibial band contracture (Fig. 2). The mean risk of progression is 15°/year; an earlier loss of walking ability corresponds with a higher rate of progression. The angle progression also depends on the balance between the sagittal and frontal planes (Oda et al., 1993; Suzuki et al., 1993). In cases of tilted pelvis and lumbar kyphosis the risk of progression is very high; in cases of double curve and preserved lumbar lordosis the risk is high; if the curve is less than 30° and the sagittal plane straight, the risk of progression is low (Fig. 3). Patients presenting a rapid curve progression are at risk of earlier death.

2. *Spinal atrophy patients* (Phillips et al., 1990; Shapiro & Specht, 1993b) have a very high risk of progression because of the very early onset of the curve. These non-walking patients have knee and hip contractures and develop a collapsing spine with important scoliosis and kyphosis. Sixty-two per cent of the curves are in the thoraco-lumbar area, 16 per cent are double curves and the other curves are thoracic or lumbar. In young patients the spine is flexible, but with age it tends to become very stiff.

3. *Congenital myopathy* (Shapiro et al., 1993a) patients are less prone to developing scoliosis. In nemaline myopathy scoliosis is infrequent but is associated with lumbar lordosis. A third of central core myopathy patients develop scoliosis similar to an idiopathic one, but the curves are very rigid and tend to have further progression after skeletal maturity.

4. In *Friedreich's ataxia* (Labelle et al., 1986) 100 per cent of patients have scoliosis of more than 10°. Thoracic hyper-

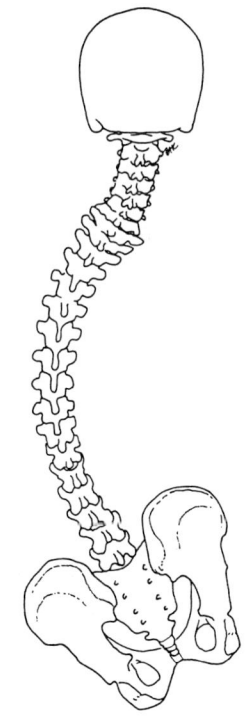

Fig. 1. Typical neuromuscular C-shaped curve with pelvic obliquity.

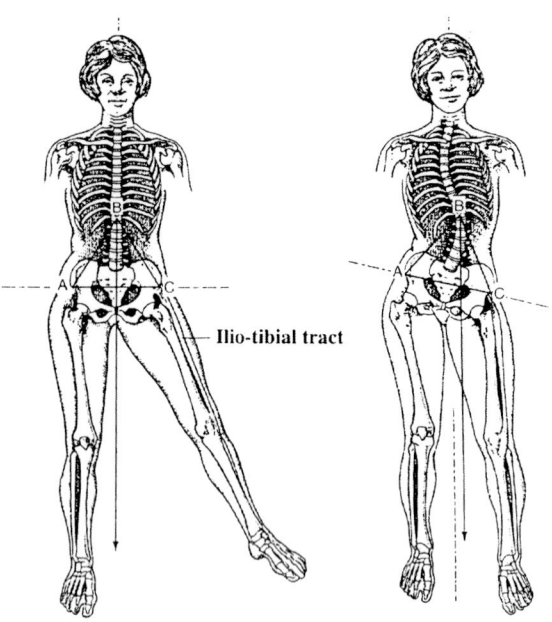

Fig. 2. Relationship between the iliotibial band and the side of the scoliosis. (Reproduced from: Cambridge, W. & Drennan, J.C. (1987): Scoliosis associated with Duchenne muscular dystrophy. J. Pediatr. Orthop., 7, 436–440.)

kyphosis is associated in 66 per cent, the progression rate of both kyphosis and scoliosis being very high if the spine deformities appear before puberty. There is no correlation between muscle weakness, ambulatory status and the risk of progression.

5. *Rett syndrome patients* (Lindström *et al.*, 1994) develop curves in 45 per cent of cases. One hundred per cent of the curves exceeding 20 per cent may progress. The C-shaped curves are associated with hyperkyphosis. Scoliosis in Rett syndrome develops at an earlier age than idiopathic forms, and its progression is more rapid.

Treatment decisions

Strategic decisions depend mainly on the diagnosis; the majority of patients are known for their neuromuscular problems before the onset of scoliosis. Global treatment aims at keeping the highest functional ability and at increasing the patient's comfort.

Functional abilities are as follows:

increasing:	walking ability
	mobility
	transfer ability
preserving:	sitting balance
	social integration
	the use of upper limbs.

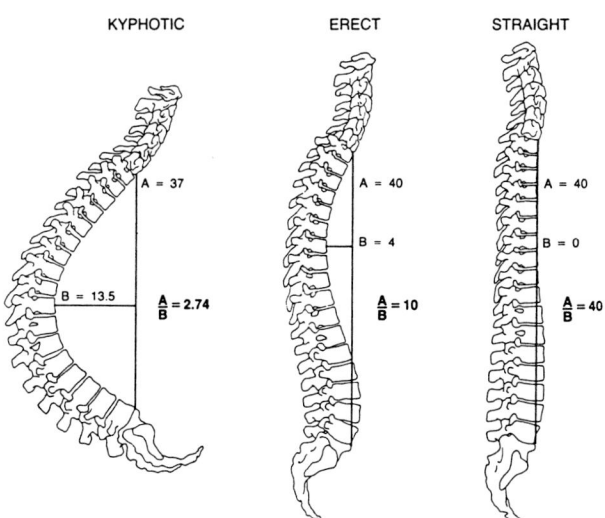

Fig. 3. Left: kyphotic deformity which represents a high risk of progression. Right: straight spine which represents a low risk of progression. The index A/B = 10 in a normal spine; lower index A/B = higher risk of progression; higher index A/B = lower risk of progression. (Reproduced from:Cambridge, W. & Drennan, J.C. (1987): Scoliosis associated with Duchenne muscular dystrophy. J. Pediatr. Orthop., 7, 436–440.)

Comfort criteria are as follows:
    avoiding: pain
                   skin sores
                   positions that interfere with care and feeding.

Screening for spinal deformities is thus mandatory for all neuromuscular patients, at all ages and not only around puberty. A complete functional examination will detect early signs of impairment which can lead to scoliosis, such as hip contracture and pelvic imbalance. The loss of walking ability and growth spurts are always correlated with higher risks of scoliosis progression.

As soon as scoliosis and/or kyphosis are detected, regular documentation of progression is organized with frontal and lateral X-rays, including the pelvis and head. This is the only method of assessing the whole function and balance of the spine unit.

Active and passive physical treatment counteracts contractures and loss of spontaneous movements, and increases compensation positioning and balance ability. The use of orthoses (leg braces, thoraco-lumbar braces, and standing devices) has more of a functional purpose than a therapeutic one. Sitting braces and adapted wheelchairs are very important for patients who have lost the ability to walk.

Brace treatment (Letts et al., 1992) is mainly performed in small curves (<20°), or in very young patients (1 year old) with flexible curves. Usually braces do not correct or control curve progression; they are indicated to increase sitting comfort or as a means of slowing down the progression while waiting for surgery in pre-puberty patients. Brace treatments can be the cause of respiratory failure, discomfort and pressure sores.

Surgical indications and techniques

Surgical correction in neuromuscular spinal deformities became popular in the 1980s. Former instrumentation and spondylodesis was followed by months in a plaster cast, and the length and magnitude of the surgical procedure were the causes of numerous complications and death (respiratory and/or cardiac failure, blood loss, infection, loss of correction).

Progress in anaesthesia and intensive care as well as the development of segmental spinal fixation allow us to perform spondylodesis with a low risk.

Nowadays indications for surgery are:

>curves with a progression of 30° in children older than 10–12 years old
>trunk collapse
>sitting imbalance
>to avoid the discomfort of a permanent brace.

Usually only posterior instrumentation is performed. Anterior release, with epiphysiodesis and/or instrumentation are performed in very young children, for very important pelvic obliquity and when posterior elements are lacking (O'Brien et al., 1992).

Pre-operative assessment includes:

>Cardiac check-up (Friedreich's and Duchenne's)
>Respiratory function (forced vital capacity 30 per cent)
>Risk of hyperthermia
>Preventive methods to limit blood loss (autotransfusion, blood recuperation)
>Ambulatory status (surgery decreases muscular strength)
>The need for hip and/or pelvic surgery in order to obtain a balanced spine
>Should the pelvis be included in the instrumentation?
>Bending films of the spine in order to choose the levels of fixation.

The surgical procedure must provide a well-balanced and stable fixation, allowing early mobilization without a brace. Modern instrumentation (Boachie-Adjei *et al.*, 1989; Broom *et al.*, 1989; Kalen *et al.*, 1992; O'Brien *et al.*, 1992; Stevens & Beard, 1989) (Luque, C-D) provides these conditions. If the pelvis is part of the curve it should be included in the fixation (Boachie-Adjei *et al.*, 1989; Stevens & Beard, 1989), but if the lumbosacral junction is balanced the instrumentation can be stopped at L5 (Stevens & Beard, 1989).

If the failure of instrumentation without arthrodesis is well accepted (Eberle *et al.*, 1988), some authors advocate the use of autologous bone graft (Zeller *et al.*, 1994), with the insertion of a tibial strut, while others (Bridewell *et al.*, 1994; Lonstein & Renshaw, 1987) propose allografts with a similar success in obtaining a good arthrodesis.

We routinely use dried crushed cancellous allograft bone without complication. During surgery, recording of the somatosensory evoked potentials is very useful for the early detection of neurological impairment (Williamson & Galasko, 1992). Prophylactic antibiotics are prescribed.

Post-operative care includes very early mobilization and respiratory re-education. Pain control is very important and epidural catheters are useful. As the loss of respiratory function is temporary, the course of the illness is not changed. Galasko *et al.* (1992) show, in their very important paper on spinal stabilization in Duchenne's muscular dystrophy, that the rate of loss of respiratory function is not changed by surgery but the death rate at 5 years after surgery is 20 per cent in operated patients and 80 per cent in non-operated ones, the quality of life of the stabilized patients being far higher.

Surgical stabilization of neuromuscular spinal deformities is nowadays a palliative, useful and widely accepted means of treatment.

Surgical indication depends on accurate diagnosis, knowledge of the natural history, and well-documented spinal deformities. Our techniques allow us to perform spinal fusions with controlled, low risks, and these procedures provide a stable and balanced spine on a horizontal pelvis.

Surgery must provide an increased quality of life and easier care; spondylodesis is only performed with the full agreement of the patient, his family and all the therapeutic team.

References

Boachie-Adjei, O., Lonstein, J.E., Winter, R.B., Koop, S., Vanden Brink, K. & Denis F.(1989): Management of neuromuscular spinal deformities with Luque segmental instrumentation. *J. Bone. & Joint Surg. [Am]* **71A,** 548–562.

Bridwell, K.H., O'Brien, M.F., Lenke, L.G., Baldus, C. & Blanke, K. (1994): Posterior spinal fusion supplemented with only allograft bone in paralytic scoliosis: does it work? *Spine* **19,** 2658–2666.

Broom, M.J., Banta, J.V. & Renshaw, T.S. (1989): Spinal fusion augmented by Luque-rod segmental instrumentation for neuromuscular scoliosis. *J. Bone & Joint Surg. [Am]* **71A,** 32–44.

Brown, J.C. & Swank, S.M. (1985): Paralytic spine deformity. In: *The pediatric spine*, eds D.S. Bradford & R.M. Hensinger, pp. 251–272. New York: Thieme Inc.

Cambridge, W. & Drennan, J.C. (1987): Scoliosis associated with Duchenne muscular dystrophy. *J. Pediatr. Orthop.* **7,** 436–440.

Daher, Y.H., Lonstein, J.E., Winter, R.B. & Moe, J.H. (1985): Spinal deformities in patients with arthrogryposis. *Spine* **10,** 609–613.

Daher, Y.H., Lonstein, J.E., Winter, R.B. & Bardford, D.S. (1986): Spinal deformities in patients with Charcot–Marie–Tooth disease. *Clin. Orthop.* **202,** 219–222.

Dearlof, W.W., Betz, R.R., Vogel, L.C., Levin, J., Clancy, M. & Steel, H.H. (1990): Scoliosis in pediatric spinal cord-injured patients. *J. Pediatr. Orthop.* **10,** 214–218.

Eberle, C.F. (1988): Failure of fixation after segmental spinal instrumentation without arthrodesis in the management of paralytic scoliosis. *J. Bone & Joint Surg. [Am]* **70A,** 696–703.

Galasko, C.S.B., Delaney, C. & Morris, P. (1992): Spinal stabilization in Duchenne muscular dystrophy. *J. Bone & Joint Surg. [Br]* **74B,** 210–214.

Kalen, V., Conklin, M.M. & Sherman, F.C. (1992): Untreated scoliosis in severe cerebral palsy. *J. Pediatr. Orthop.* **12,** 337–340.

Labelle, H., Tohmé, S., Duhaime, M. & Allard, P. (1986): Natural history of scoliosis in Friedreich's ataxia. *J. Bone & Joint Surg. [Am]* **68A,** 564–572.

Letts, M., Rathbone, D., Yamashita, T., Nichil, B. & Keeler, A.(1992): Soft Boston orthosis in management of neuromuscular scoliosis: a preliminary report. *J. Pediatr. Orthop.* **12,** 470–474.

Lindström, J., Stockland, E. & Hagberg, B.(1994): Scoliosis in Rett syndrome. *Spine* **19,** 1632–1635.

Lonstein, J.E. & Renshaw, T.S. (1987): Neuromuscular spine deformities. In: *Instructional Course Lectures,* Vol. 36, pp. 285–304. Washington DC: American Academy of Orthopaedic Surgeons.

Mubarak, S.J., Morin, W.D. & Leach, J. (1993): Spinal fusion in Duchenne muscular dystrophy – fixation and fusion to the pelvis. *J. Pediatr. Orthop.* **13,** 752–757.

O'Brien, T., Akmajian, J., Ogin, G. & Eilert, R. (1992): Comparison of one-stage versus two-stage anterior/posterior spinal fusion for neuromuscular scoliosis. *J. Pediatr. Orthop.* **12,** 610–615.

Oda, T., Shimizu, N., Vonenobu, K., Ono, K., Nabeshima, T. & Kyoh, S. (1993): Longitudinal study of spinal deformity in Duchenne muscular dystrophy. *J. Pediatr. Orthop.* **13,** 478–488.

Phillips, D.P., Roye, D.P., Farcy, J-P., Lett, A. & Shelton, Y.A. (1990): Surgical treatment of scoliosis in a spinal atrophy population. *Spine* **15,** 942–945.

Rinsky, L.A. (1990): Surgery of spinal deformity in cerebral palsy. *Clin. Orthop.* **253,** 100–109.

Shapiro, F. & Specht, L. (1993a): The diagnosis and orthopaedic treatment of inherited muscular diseases of childhood. *J. Bone & Joint Surg. [Am]* **75A,** 439–454.

Shapiro, F. & Specht, L. (1993b): The diagnosis and orthopaedic treatment of childhood spinal atrophy, peripheral neuropathy, Friedreich's ataxia and arthrogryposis. *J. Bone & Joint Surg. [Am]* **75A,** 1699–1714.

Smith, A.D., Koreska, J. & Moseley, C.F. (1989): Progression of scoliosis in Duchenne muscular dystrophy. *J. Bone & Joint Surg. [Am]* **71A,** 1066–1074.

Smith, R.M. & Emans, J.B. (1992): Sitting balance in spinal deformities. *Spine* **17,** 1103–1109.

Stagnara, P. (1985): *Les déformations du rachis*, pp. 124–142. Paris, Masson.

Stevens, D.B. & Beard, C. (1989): Segmental spinal instrumentation for neuromuscular spinal deformity. *Clin. Orthop.* **242,** 164–168.

Suzuki, S., Kasahara, Y., Yamamoto, S., Seto, Y., Fukurawa, K. & Nishino Y. (1993): Three-dimensional spinal deformity in scoliosis associated with cerebral palsy and progressive muscular dystrophy. *Spine* **18,** 2290–2294.

Williamson, J.B. & Galasko, C.S.B. (1992): Spinal cord monitoring during operative correction of neuromuscular scoliosis. *J. Bone & Joint Surg. [Am]* **74B,** 870–872.

Zeller, R., Ghanem, I., Miladi, L. & Dubousset, J. (1994): Posterior spinal fusion in neuromuscular scoliosis using a tibial strut graft. *Spine* **19,** 1628–1631.

Chapter 12

Respiratory pathophysiological bases for mechanical ventilation in neuromuscular diseases

Isa Cerveri, Francesco Fanfulla and Maria Cristina Zoia

Institute of Respiratory Diseases, Policlinico San Matteo, Piazzale Golgi, 27100 Pavia, Italy

Summary

Advances in knowledge about the respiratory changes and mechanisms of development of respiratory failure in many neuromuscular diseases have led to an improved rationalization of the therapeutic strategies; however, many aspects, particularly those concerning ventilatory therapy, remain to be clarified. Because of the extreme heterogeneity of the neuromuscular diseases, the changes in respiratory failure and their course over time have, in part, different characteristics leading to different respiratory pathophysiological pictures. In general, a whole series of pathological events whose evolution over time causes a progressive worsening of respiratory function are based on two fundamental changes: the deficits in the strength of skeletal respiratory muscles and of those of the thoracic cage. These alterations generate progressive reduction of pulmonary volumes and changes in respiratory mechanics, so that a vicious circle is created whose final result is an increased resistive load, which is sustained by an ever less adequate pump system.

In the treatment of manifest respiratory failure, there is now good agreement in the literature on the inclusion criteria defined as necessary for mechanical ventilation of hypercapnic patients. There does not seem to be room, however, for the so-called 'preventive' ventilation proposed in the past to delay the onset of respiratory failure. In this context we have suggested the possible identification of a set of patients who could benefit from mechanical ventilation at a particular point in the natural evolution of their disease towards chronic respiratory failure before it becomes manifest. The results of our study suggest that the presence of nocturnal hypoventilation, even in the absence of daytime alterations in gas exchange, should be considered as an inclusion criterion for mechanical ventilation.

The natural history of many neuromuscular diseases is characterized by the development of respiratory failure which is also the major cause of death. In the past, the treatment of chronic respiratory failure in these diseases was almost entirely reserved for patients already extremely compromised, and was based exclusively on empirical criteria. At present, advances in knowledge about the respiratory changes and mechanisms of development of respiratory failure have led to an improved rationalization of the therapeutic strategies, although many aspects remain to be clarified, particularly those concerning ventilatory therapy. Because of the extreme heterogeneity of these pathologies, changes in respiratory failure and their course over time have, in part, different characteristics and it is not possible to describe a single pathophysiological picture. This is even more the case in the forms that occur in growing patients in whom the pathological processes affecting the thoracopulmonary system are influenced by the dynamics of growth. Consequently, therapeutic indications must also be evaluated from pathology to pathology; in particular, mechanical ventilation is a therapeutic strategy for which, at present, reasonably well-controlled results have been obtained from fairly homogeneous populations only in Duchenne's muscular dystrophy (DMD). For this reason, this chapter refers only to this disease, although many of the considerations could be extended to other pathologies. There is one extremely important point that needs emphasis: the complex evaluation necessary to start ventilatory therapy and all the choices which need to be made to control and delay the onset of respiratory failure require total involvement by the patient in order to be achieved as early as possible. The progressive changes in respiratory function must be carefully evaluated and subsequently the patient and family must be prepared for the possibility of recourse to a ventilatory prosthesis. This must be a choice made on the basis of a careful evaluation of the cost–benefit ratio and it is vital not to become faced, as has often happened in the past, by situations of acute respiratory emergency, that were not previously assessed from a pulmonary point of view and thus demand urgent decisions which cannot be reflected upon as is necessary. It is important to remember that respiratory symptomatology often does not correlate with the degree of respiratory involvement in DMD and likewise for many other myopathies: so careful monitoring of respiratory function must be carried out over time, in addition to monitoring of the symptoms (Lynn et al., 1994).

Pathophysiological bases

Table 1 shows the more salient changes in respiratory mechanics in DMD. A whole series of pathological events whose evolution over time causes a progressive worsening of respiratory function is based on two fundamental changes: the deficits in strength of the skeletal respiratory muscles and of those of the thoracic cage.

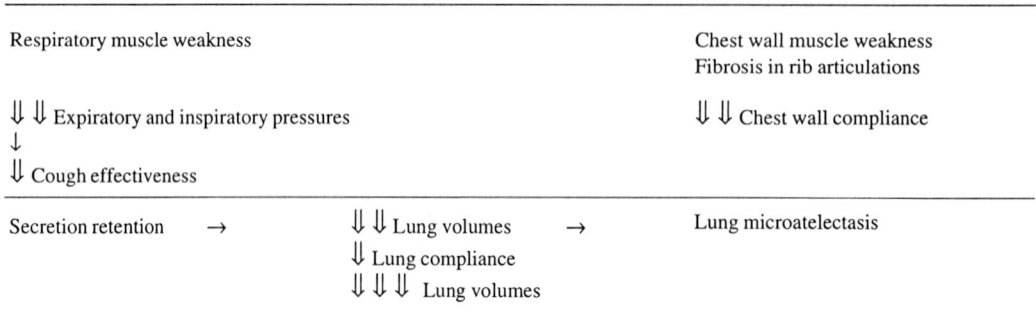

Table 1. Respiratory mechanics in DMD

Respiratory muscle weakness		Chest wall muscle weakness
		Fibrosis in rib articulations
⇓⇓ Expiratory and inspiratory pressures ↓		⇓⇓ Chest wall compliance
⇓ Cough effectiveness		
Secretion retention →	⇓⇓ Lung volumes → ⇓ Lung compliance ⇓⇓⇓ Lung volumes	Lung microatelectasis

The decrease in respiratory muscle strength causes a reduction in maximal respiratory pressures in the mouth; the expiratory pressure is more altered than the inspiratory, and this seems to demonstrate a greater involvement of the abdominal muscles with respect to the major inspiratory muscle, that is, the diaphragm.

The reduction in the inspiratory pressure creates a decreased ability to expectorate with a consequent increase in retention of secretions and thus a further decrease in lung volume.

However, marked scoliosis and fibrotic retraction of ligamentous and articular structures of the thoracic cage can also result in a further decrease in lung volumes by means of the consequent increase in the rigidity of the system and reduction in the thoracic compliance. The onset of microatelectasis due to the progressive reduction in mobility of the entire thoracopulmonary system further aggravates the respiratory deficit, completing the vicious circle. The final result is that of an increased resistive load sustained by an ever less adequate pump system compromised by a progressive disease.

Chapter 12 Respiratory pathophysiological bases

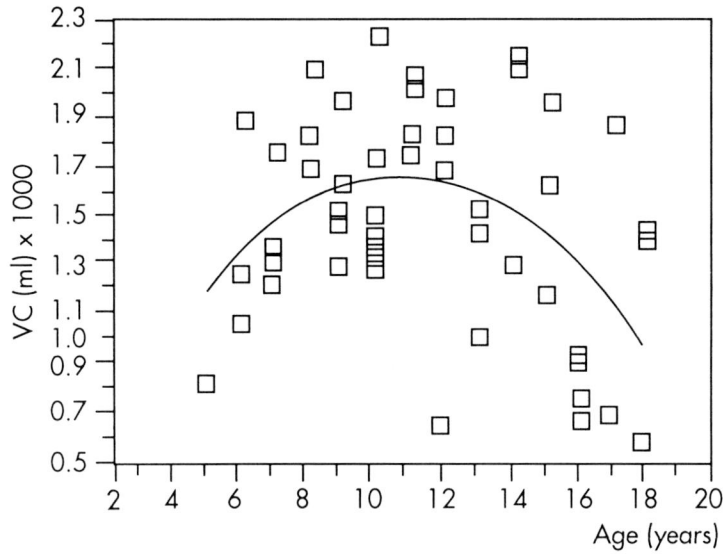

Fig. 1. Cross-sectional study of the correlation between vital capacity (VC) and age in 26 patients with DMD.

Fig. 1 illustrates the trend in vital capacity (VC) with age, recorded in a cross-sectional study in our patients which confirms the known trend described by Rideau & Delaubier (1988): an initial increase in accordance with body growth, a second plateau phase in which, despite body growth, the value of the parameter tends to remain stable, and finally the phase of progressive decrease which is estimated to be about 200–250 ml per year.

Fig. 2 reports a study by De Troyer et al. (1980) showing the relationship between respiratory muscle strength and vital capacity. It is clear that the reduction in VC is greater than expected from the degree of muscle weakness, confirming the influence of the changes associated with the alteration in thoracopulmonary compliance (in particular, scoliosis and microatelectasis).

The pattern of breathing under baseline conditions also tends to change progressively, compared to the normal subject; it becomes fast and shallow due to the reduction in tidal volume and increase in respiratory frequency (Fig. 3). This pattern seems to be adopted strategically by these patients because of the progressive weakness of the respiratory muscles; it seems to be the pattern which requires the least work and is thus the least tiring.

By contrast with many other neuromuscular diseases, for example Steinert's dystrophy, significant changes in the central regulation of breathing are not present in DMD. The progression of the changes in respiratory mechanics makes the patients, at around 20 years old, inexorably slide towards a picture of recognized chronic alveolar hypoventilation characterized by a reduction in arterial blood PaO_2 and an increase in $PaCO_2$. Only a weak relationship between the degree of muscle weakness and the level of hypercapnia has been observed, and this confirms the involvement of other factors such as changes in the static mechanical properties of the respiratory system, onset of respiratory muscle fatigue and the different responses of the respiratory centres to changes in the gases (Estenne, 1991). Sometimes, when the respiratory equilibrium is already precarious, an

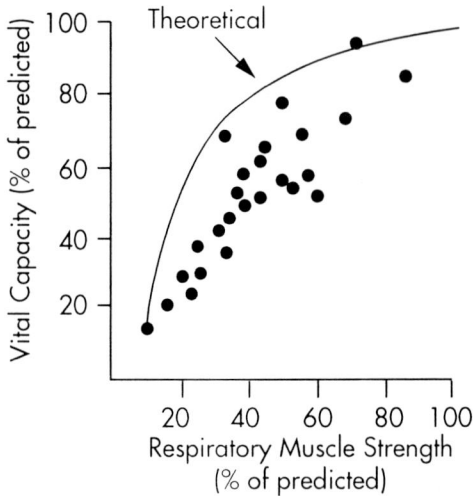

Fig. 2. Respiratory muscle strength and vital capacity in DMD.

episode of acute bronchial inflammation with further stagnation of secretions is sufficient to cause a dramatic picture of acute respiratory failure which necessitates the use of mechanical ventilation.

There is generally agreement in the literature (Unterborn & Hill, 1994; Vianello et al., 1994; Hill, 1994) on the inclusion criteria defined as necessary for ventilation of hypercapnic patients. There does not seem to be room, however – at least at present following the negative results reported in the recent important study by Raphael et al. (1994) – for the so-called 'preventive' ventilation proposed in the past with the aim of delaying the onset of respiratory failure.

In this context we have, in the past, studied the possibility of identifying a set of patients who could benefit from mechanical ventilation at a particular point in the natural evolution of their disease towards chronic respiratory failure, before it becomes manifest. That is, we set ourselves the task of identifying the most opportune time to begin ventilation therapy. The studies on respiratory disorders during sleep in these patients which Manni et al. (1989, 1991) and other groups (Smith et al., 1988) have conducted over the years have suggested that this moment is represented by the presence of nocturnal hypoventilation without alterations in gas exchange during wakefulness, thus in patients not yet in imperative need of ventilation.

Table 2. Factors conditioning $HbSaO_2$ reductions during sleep in DMD

During wakefulness	During sleep
Respiratory muscle weakness + severe scoliosis ⇓	⇓⇓ (REM phase)
Marked and progressive reduction of pulmonary volumes ⇓	⇓⇓ FRC (supine position)
Rapid shallow breathing	⇓⇓ Breathing pattern irregularities in REM phase
Obesity	OSA (obstructive sleep apnoea)

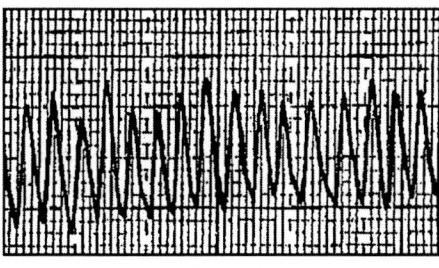

Normal
(L.S., 18 years old)

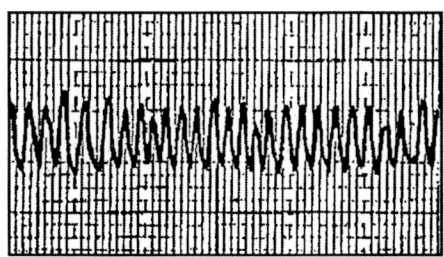

Rapid and shallow
(G.B., 18 years old – DMD)

Fig. 3. Pattern of breathing.

The factors conditioning the fall in arterial haemoglobin oxygen saturation ($HbSaO_2$) during nocturnal sleep in DMD are illustrated in Table 2. In brief, the nocturnal deterioration can be attributed to upsetting the already precarious respiratory equilibrium during wakefulness; during sleep, changes in respiratory mechanics and control mechanisms of breathing which are linked to the physiological characteristics of sleep (reduction in the functional residual capacity due to the supine position, intercostal muscle hypotonia and irregularity of the breathing pattern in the REM phase) are superimposed on the changes previously described as present during wakefulness. Furthermore, obesity is a frequent characteristic of these patients.

Thus, a nocturnal polysomnographic study was set up, with a follow-up after 2 years of 9 patients (mean age 16.2 years, range 10–20) whose characteristics are reported in Table 3. As can be seen, respiratory function and gas exchange, both at the control baseline and after 2 years, were well conserved, despite registering the expected well-known decline in the respiratory functional and blood-gas parameters.

Table 3. Respiratory function during wakefulness baseline and after 2 years' follow-up

	Baseline	2 years follow-up
VC (lt)	1.7 (1.3–2.1)	1.4 (0.6–1.9)
FRC (lt)	1.7 (1.3–4.0)	1.5 (1.3–3.3)
PaO_2 (mmHg)	88.4 (83–94)	85 (73–96)
$PaCO_2$ (mmHg)	40 (37–45)	40.3 (38–44)

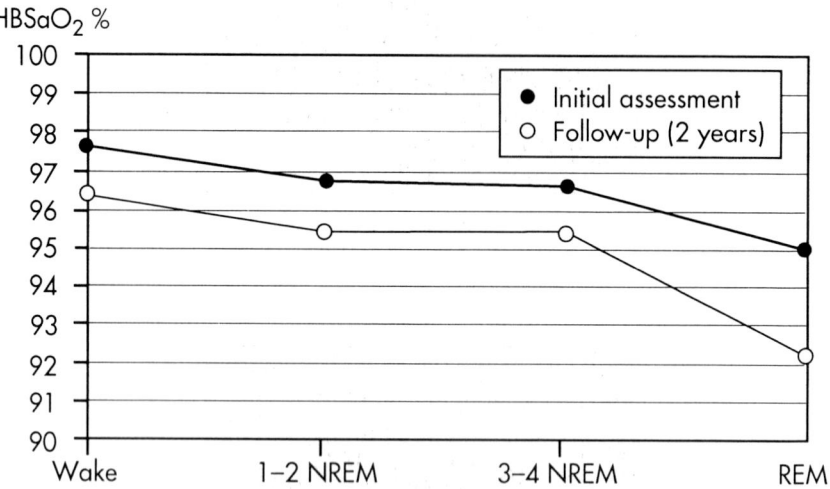

Fig. 4. HbSaO$_2$: Mean values during sleep in DMD (P < 0.05).

Fig. 4 shows the mean values of HbSaO$_2$ in the various phases of sleep at baseline and at the 2-year follow-up. A drop in the average values of HbSaO$_2$ can be noted in the REM phase at both evaluations, but with a statistically significant worsening at the assessment after 2 years.

Fig. 5 shows the drop in HbSaO$_2$ for each patient, with the HbSaO$_2$ at the first measurement being under 90 per cent for four patients; these patients had deteriorated clearly by the second control and a further two patients had saturations less than 90 per cent. It can be seen from Table 4 that the deteriorating trend of nocturnal HbSaO$_2$ tended to worsen in parallel with the respiratory function during wakefulness. The important point is, however, that in the group of subjects defined as desaturators (HbSaO$_2$ < 90 per cent) the VC and the PaO$_2$ decreased much more rapidly at the 2-year control than in the others.

Table 4. Daytime respiratory function baseline and after 2 years' follow-up in patients with and without nocturnal desaturation at baseline

	Desaturators	Non-desaturators
VC–baseline (lt)	1.712 ± 0.241	1.786 ± 0.326
VC–2 years (lt)	1.224 ± 0.327	1.661 ± 0.390
PaO$_2$–baseline (mmHg)	89.3 ± 4.8	87.7 ± 4.92
PeO$_2$–2 years (mmHg)	83.0 ± 6.32	85.5 ± 8.6

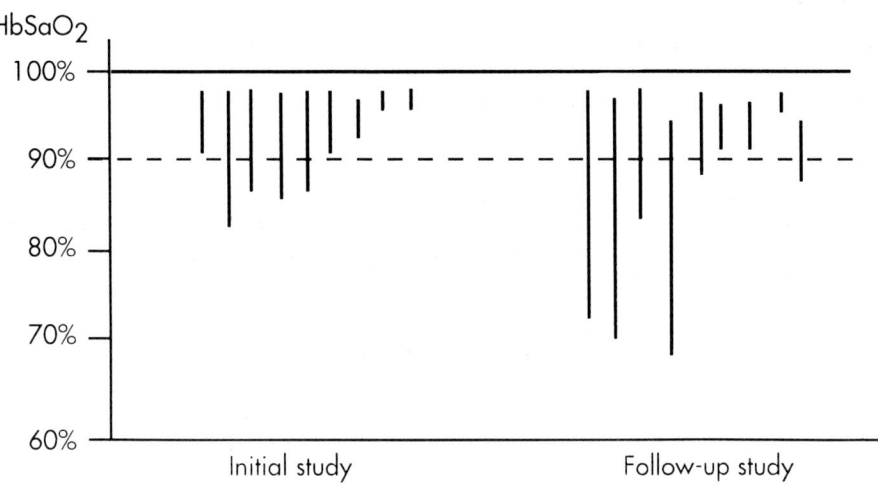

Fig. 5. Lowest HbSaO$_2$ values during sleep for each patient.

Sleep-disordered breathing as a criterion for mechanical ventilation

In the light of these results, it was decided to conduct a subsequent study with this important question: do respiratory disorders during sleep represent a criterion for mechanical ventilation? From another perspective, Hill (1993) suggested that preventing nocturnal hypoventilation with the possible resetting of the sensitivity to CO_2 of the respiratory centres could be the most important mechanism of mechanical ventilation.

In order to check the most appropriate time to start mechanical ventilation in DMD we conducted a 2-year follow-up study of 13 patients in an advanced stage of the disease who were offered nocturnal non-invasive pressure support ventilation via a nasal mask (Bi-PAP; Respironics). All patients enrolled into the study satisfied the following inclusion criteria:

1. SaO_2 drops, defined as a reduction in SaO_2 to under 90 per cent, the overall duration of which had to be longer than at least 10 per cent of the time in bed (TB – with $SaO_2 < 90$ per cent); and at least one of the following: 2. VC reduced by more than 20 per cent in the previous 6 months; 3. Daytime symptoms of sleep-disordered breathing (SDB).

Study design

All the patients enrolled in the study underwent analysis of their respiratory function while awake (spirometry, maximal respiratory pressure at the mouth, blood-gas analysis) and during sleep (overnight SaO_2 monitoring). All the patients were admitted to hospital for at least 3 days to become accustomed to the ventilator. The setting of the ventilation parameters was performed after continuous monitoring of the patient's breathing pattern (with Respitrace) and the SaO_2 value; the lower values of inspiratory (IPAP) and expiratory (EPAP) positive pressures which allowed the best increase in tidal volume and correction of the episodes of nocturnal desaturation were chosen. In addition, in order to avoid the appearance of respiratory alkalosis, the patients underwent blood gas analyses at baseline and during ventilation. Furthermore, the study protocol called for the measurement of the same parameters after 1 and 2 years; in particular, samples for blood-gas analysis were taken at least 3 h after ending ventilatory treatment.

Study population

Initially 13 patients were enrolled, but two of these refused ventilator treatment. Of the remaining 11, one died 13 months after the start of the study from acute respiratory failure and another was admitted to hospital with pneumonia at the time of the 2-year control.

Control group

Eight DMD patients were enrolled as the control group. Seven completed the study and the other required mechanical ventilation. These subjects were younger than the treated patients and their respiratory functions were less compromised. Table 5 reports the demographics and baseline respiratory data of the patients and the control subjects.

Table 5. Demography and respiratory function at entry into the study for treated patients and controls (mean values and range)

	Age (years)	VC (ml)	PaO$_2$ (mmHg)	PaCO$_2$ (mmHg)	TB < 90% (%)
NPSV patients	18–25 (15–22)	75.2 (430–1308)	78 (70–87.8)	44.3 (36.3–48.5)	31.6 (16.6–65)
Controls	16.4 (10–21)	1445 (990–2011)	85.7 (78–94)	42.5 (39–48)	4.21 (2.6–7)

Results

None of the patients treated with mechanical ventilation required a change in the ventilatory parameters selected, as demonstrated by the disappearance of the episodes of nocturnal desaturation.

Table 6 reports respiratory data from the patients and the control subjects at the 2-year follow-up. Both ventilated patients and control subjects showed a progressive decline in VC, although there is a marked dispersion of data. A statistically significant difference was observed between baseline and follow-up VC values both in the ventilated and control patients ($P = 0.003$ and $P = 0.03$ respectively). No statistically significant difference was observed between baseline and follow-up blood-gas values either in the treated or control group. Treated patients showed a slight increase in PaO$_2$ while the control patients had a slight decrease.

The control group showed a more rapid, statistically significant decline in VC compared to the ventilated patients (–214.4 ml/year ± 115 versus –79.1 ml/year ± 25, $P = 0.02$).

Table 6. Respiratory function after 2 years' follow-up of treated patients and controls (mean values and range)

	VC (ml)	PaO$_2$ (mmHg)	PaCO$_2$ (mmHg)	TB < 90% (%)
NPSV patients	594.3 (280–1090)	81.7 (73–87.8)	45.5 (37–55)	0.6 (0–1.2)
Controls	1017 (450–1471)	83 (74–93)	42.5 (39–48)	8.7 (3.15)

Conclusions

Our results indicate that non-invasive nocturnal ventilation with Bi-PAP is effective in normalizing gas exchange during sleep. Furthermore, these patients, despite their decline in ventilatory function shown by the reduction in VC, maintain adequate oxygenation during the day without increases in carbon dioxide.

Comparing the trend of respiratory function in a control group, unfortunately not perfectly matched, would seem to show a slowing in the rate of decrease of VC. Thus, this study suggests that patients affected by advanced DMD, with pronounced episodes of nocturnal desaturation, while not fulfilling criteria for imperative ventilatory therapy, could be treated with benefit in terms of preserving respiratory residual capacity with 'elective' nocturnal ventilation.

References

De Troyer, A., Barenstein, S. & Cadier, R. (1980): Analysis of lung volume restriction in patients with respiratory muscle weakness. *Thorax* **35**, 603–607.

De Troyer, A. & Pride, N.B. (1986): The respiratory system in neuromuscular disorders. In: *The thorax*, part B, eds C. Roussos & P.T. Macklem, pp. 1089–1121. New York: Marcel Dekker.

Estenne, M. (1991): Pathophysiology of ventilatory failure in patients with neuromyopathies. In: *Ventilatory failure*, eds. D.J. Marini & C. Roussos, pp. 240–254. Berlin, Heidelberg: Springer Verlag.

Hill, N.S. (1994): Noninvasive positive pressure ventilation in neuromuscular disease: enough is enough. *Chest* **105**, 337–338.

Hill, N.S. (1993): Noninvasive ventilation: does it work, for whom, and how? *Am. Rev. Respir. Dis.* **147**, 1050–1055.

Lynn, D.J., Woda, R.P. & Mendell, J.R. (1994): Respiratory dysfunction in muscular dystrophy and other myopathies. In: *Clinics in chest medicine*, eds B.L. Fanfurg & L. Sicilian, pp. 661–674. Philadelphia: W.B. Saunders.

Smith, P.E.M., Galverly, P.M.A. & Edwards, R.H.T. (1988): Hypoxemia during sleep in Duchenne muscular dystrophy. *Am. Rev. Respir. Dis.* **137**, 884.

Manni, R., Ottolini, A., Cerveri, I., Bruschi, C., Zoia, M.C., Lanzi, G. & Tartara A. (1989): Breathing patterns and $HbSaO_2$ changes during nocturnal sleep in patients with Duchenne muscular dystrophy. *J. Neurol.* **23B**, 391–394.

Manni, R., Zucca, C., Galimberti, C., Ottolini, A., Cerveri, I., Bruschi, C., Zoia, M.C., Lanzi, G. & Tartara, A. (1991): Nocturnal sleep and oxygen balance in Duchenne muscular dystrophy: A clinical and polygraphic 2-year follow-up study. *Eur. Arch. Psychiatry Clin. Neurosci.* **240**, 255–257.

Raphael, J.C., Chevret, S., Chastang, C. & Bouvet, F. (1994): Randomised trial of preventive nasal ventilation in Duchenne muscular dystrophy. *Lancet* **343**, 1600–1604.

Rideau, J. & Delaubier, A. (1988): Management of respiratory neuromuscular weakness. *Muscle Nerve* **11**, 407–408.

Unterborn, J.N. & Hill, N.S. (1994): Options for mechanical ventilation in neuromuscular diseases. In: *Clinics of chest medicine*, eds. B.L. Fanburg & L. Sicilian, pp. 765–781. Philadelphia: W.B. Saunders.

Vianello, A., Bevilacqua, M., Selvador, V., Cardaioli, C. & Vincenti, E. (1994): Long-term nasal intermittent positive pressure ventilation in advanced Duchenne muscular dystrophy. *Chest* **105**, 446–448.

Chapter 13

Home mechanical ventilation and Duchenne's muscular dystrophy

Jean-Claude Raphael

Service de Réanimation Médicale, Hôpitaux de Paris, 104 boulevard R. Poincaré, 92380 Garches, France

Summary

Duchenne's muscular dystrophy is the most frequent of muscular dystrophies. Its evolution is ineluctably fatal with the onset of cardiac and/or respiratory insufficiency. Attitudes towards respiratory treatment are controversial in the literature. Nevertheless, the few available series, all retrospective, show that home mechanical ventilation can be organized, raising the survival rate. However, its indications and the optimal ventilation technique are not defined. That is why two multicentric prospective studies were initiated. Imperative ventilation has the goal of palliating respiratory muscle paralysis. The preliminary results show that intermittent positive pressure by tracheotomy is more efficient than non-invasive methods. Preventive ventilation has the goal of reducing the aggravation of the respiratory handicap. The results of a randomized study show that, paradoxically, the mortality risk is greater within the ventilated group than in the control group. The fall in vital capacity is identical in both groups. The indication for imperative mechanical home ventilation must be decided in a stable state with a vital capacity of less than 20 per cent of the theoretical value and/or the advent of hypercapnia greater than 45 mmHg. Non-invasive ventilation system can, at first intention, be proposed, but will sooner or later have to be replaced by tracheotomy.

Duchenne's muscular dystrophy is the most frequent of the childhood muscular dystrophies. It affects one male infant in 5000 births, and its prevalence is estimated to be 3/100 000. It follows a stereotyped evolution: the first signs of the deficit appear between 2 and 3 years of age, and the ability to walk is lost between 10 and 12 years. In addition to paralysis of the limbs and the trunk there is paralysis of the respiratory muscles, in which the severity is correlated with the extent of the motor handicap (Inkley et al., 1974). The reduction in vital capacity becomes perceptible beginning at age 12, and worsens progressively. Blood-gas abnormalities appear later; the presence of hypercapnia is a particularly adverse sign. Death occurs at about 20 years old from respiratory or cardiac insufficiency.

Although therapeutic abstention in treating the respiratory handicap has been suggested, during the last 20 years some groups have proposed ventilatory assistance in a non-hospital setting. This requires a specialized organization and precise criteria both in the decision to undertake ventilation and in the choice of technique utilized.

The goal of this study is to present the various results of ventilation that have been observed, mainly in terms of survival and quality of life. After a review of the literature, we will describe the results of the French Multicentric Duchenne Muscular Dystrophy Study Group which was set up in France in 1985, and we will present the first results that have been obtained.

Review of the literature

In the evaluation of mechanical ventilation in patients with Duchenne's muscular dystrophy, three types of studies may be distinguished schematically: (i) studies on survival over several years in severely affected patients, (ii) studies over a shorter time period which evaluate a ventilatory technique using blood-gas criteria, and (iii) studies based on the early use of mechanical ventilation.

Table 1 summarizes the principal studies of the first type which have been carried out over the last 10 years. It can be seen that the mean survival varies from 5 to 10 years, which demonstrates the value of utilizing home mechanical ventilation in this disease. The most common indication for initiating ventilation is the appearance of hypercapnia of varying degrees, depending on the authors. Nevertheless, these studies are all retrospective, the means of ventilation used was very diverse, and the patients form a highly selected group in the sense that there is a large disproportion between the prevalence of the disorder and the number of patients included in the studies. The most important question seems to be the choice between two types of techniques: (i) non-invasive techniques including intermittent positive pressure ventilation (IPPV) applied by different methods (mouth, nose, abdominal compression), or intermittent negative perithoracic pressure ventilation (INPV) (cuirass, iron lung) and (ii) tracheotomy, an invasive technique which, for some authors, represents the safest technique when the vital capacity becomes very low (Baydur et al., 1990).

Table 1. Survival in Duchenne's muscular dystrophy treated with home ventilation

Authors	Number of subjects	Indications	Ventilation techniques	Average survival
Alexander et al. (1979)	n = 10	Hypercapnia	Non-invasive Positive pressure by mouth Rocking bed. Cuirass Abdominal compression	4 years
Bach et al. (1987b)	n = 31	Hypercapnia VC < 25 %	Positive pressure by mouth Iron lung Tracheotomy in case of failure	10 years
Baydur et al. (1990)	n = 17	Hypercapnia VC < 25 %	Positive pressure by mouth or nose, iron lung or cuirass Tracheotomy in case of failure or if VC below 300 ml	8 years
Curran & Colbert (1989)	n = 23	Hypercapnia	Positive pressure by mouth and iron lung Tracheotomy in case of failure.	6 years

This debate over non-invasive versus invasive techniques is encountered in studies of the second type which are short-term evaluations of either the efficacy of nasal ventilation used alone (Segall 1988; Heckmatt et al., 1990), or the combination of several non-invasive techniques which may be followed by tracheotomy in the case of failure (Mohr & Hill, 1990). In these studies, the end point used to judge the efficiency of ventilation is the disappearance of hypercapnia. From Mohr & Hill's study (1990) it is clear that this result cannot be explained by an improvement in mechanical respiratory performance which continues to deteriorate, but by a progressive increase in the daily duration of mechanical ventilation.

Some authors recommend the early use of IPPV by nasal mask at night. In fact, the first proposed use of NIPPV was for Duchenne's muscular dystrophy (Rideau, 1986, 1987; Rideau & Delaubier, 1988; Delaubier et al., 1987), and it was later extended to other pathological conditions, mainly neuromuscular disorders or to patients affected by sleep apnoea with nocturnal desaturation due to various ætiologies (Baydur, 1990; Segall, 1988; Heckmatt et al., 1990; Bach et al., 1987a; Bach & Alba, 1990; Caroll & Branthwaite, 1988; Leger et al., 1989; Ellis et al., 1987; Kerby et al., 1987).

Arguments in favour of early initiation of mechanical ventilation using a nasal mask (NIPPV) are a smaller than expected decrease in vital capacity (Delaubier et al., 1987; Granata et al., 1989), or a smaller decrease in both vital capacity and deaths (5 per cent versus 50 per cent) in 20 patients treated in this way compared with 20 controls; there was however no randomization in this latter study, and the inclusion criteria were not indicated (Delaubier et al., 1987).

In the preceding studies, the effect of ventilation on the quality of life was not considered systematically. Social or even professional reinsertion was frequently mentioned, however. In one study, quality of life was used as the end point (Bach et al., 1991), in 82 Duchenne's muscular dystrophy patients who were dependent on a mechanical ventilation technique. The clearest result of this work is that the percentage of dissatisfaction in these patients (12 per cent) is not significantly different from that in the general population (7 per cent), or in the health professionals who care for these patients (9 per cent). This percentage was not influenced by the type of ventilation (invasive or non-invasive), and satisfaction was higher in patients living at home than in institutionalized subjects. The other important result of this study is that the health professionals have a more pessimistic view about the quality of life of the patients in their care than the patients themselves. This is probably one of the explanations for the fact that the number of Duchenne's muscular dystrophy patients managed in this way in the world remains small.

Multicentric group evaluation of home ventilation techniques in Duchenne's muscular dystrophy

The absence of a consensus on the indications for home ventilation which has already been noted in the literature (Smith et al., 1988; Heckmatt, 1987) undoubtedly explains why different physicians are led to make different decisions (Colbert & Schock, 1985; Raphael, et al., 1986). This only contributes to the anguish of the patients and their families wishing to have the most accurate information possible before making a decision (Gilgoff et al., 1989; Miller et al., 1988). The difficulties involved in explaining the indications for mechanical ventilation in such an incapacitating disease with an inevitably fatal outcome are understandable. Other subacute or chronic neuromuscular diseases of children and adults elicit the same problems (Raphael et al., 1987). In addition to the ethical and logistic problems in the management of these patients, the lack of a prospective evaluation of the goals, effectiveness, morbidity, and cost of the various techniques of home mechanical ventilation explains the large differences in treatment strategy that are observed. It is therefore of fundamental importance to try to rationalize the indications for home mechanical ventilation in these disorders. Since Duchenne's muscular dystrophy is the most frequent myopathy of children and is easy to diagnose, it seemed logical to give priority to a study of this disease. With the support of the AFM (Association Française contre les Myopathies, the French Muscular Dystrophy Association), a cooperative group was created in 1985 to define the indications for home mechanical ventilation in Duchenne's muscular dystrophy. Two types of ventilation were defined: imperative ventilation and preventive ventilation (Raphael, 1987; Raphael et al., 1992a, b), which led to the designing of two studies.

Imperative ventilation

The goals of imperative ventilation are to compensate for paralysis of the respiratory muscles and to increase survival. Since this ventilation is organized in a non-hospital setting, one can hope that the quality of life will at least be preserved and possibly improved due to the disappearance of signs of respiratory insufficiency.

Nevertheless, initiating this type of ventilation depends on a certain number of prerequisites. The patient and his family must not only be in agreement with the principle of this ventilation, but moreover, must be willing to participate actively in its implementation. Home ventilation represents a considerable constraint, even in France where regional associations for respiratory insufficiency facilitate discharge from hospital and take care of the financing of the material (ventilator, aspiration apparatus, oxygen, cannulas etc.). Furthermore, it is essential that the decision to ventilate be made when the patient is in a stable state, and not during an episode of acute decompensation. This requires informing the patients, but also the physicians who too often underestimate the gravity of the respiratory handicap of these patients. Measurement of vital capacity and blood gases are simple elements of surveillance which are frequently not carried out. A decision to ventilate which is made during an acute episode with no knowledge of the basic physiological parameters causes major problems in the later discharge of the patient from hospital to home: hospitalization in critical care will be long, and weaning from the ventilator will be difficult. A conflict may arise between the patient, his or her family, and the critical care team. The patients and their families will not understand why they were not properly informed and the critical care team, because of a lack of precise information, will have trouble responding to the inevitable questions about prognosis that they will be asked.

It should be possible to resolve these questions. One solution, for example, would be to establish a preliminary dialogue between the patient, his attending physician(s), and the critical care team which will be in charge of possible decisions regarding ventilation and follow-up. The complexity of the health care system in France before 1985 made this solution quasi-impossible because the physicians involved were all different. The attending physicians were either general practitioners, or rehabilitation specialists who were not up-to-date in ventilation techniques. On the other hand, the critical care specialists were familiar with ventilation techniques but did not necessarily know about neuromuscular diseases or the constraints of home ventilation. One of the first positive consequences of the creation of the multicentric and multidisciplinary group was incontestably the improvement of communication between these different specialists. This group made it possible to identify teams which were capable of making 'good decisions' and organizing follow up. Indeed, it is very important for the prescriber to understand the impact of his decision on the subsequent management of the patient. The only solution is to organize an exhaustive and prospective follow up for the study population and to analyse the results as a function of the decision made.

The prospective multicentric study on so-called imperative ventilation involved establishing a prospective management scheme for at least 200 Duchenne's muscular dystrophy patients who had a respiratory handicap that was sufficiently severe to serve as an indication for proposing home mechanical ventilation. Six indication criteria were defined, of which the first three were evaluated during a steady state (Table 2) and three methods of ventilation were possible: nasal mask, tracheotomy, or abdominal compression. The choice of techniques could not be made randomly, but was based on a pre-established decision scheme (Table 2) which favoured non-invasive methods at first, reserving tracheotomy for cases in which other techniques failed. Nevertheless, tracheotomy could be proposed as the first measure for severely ill patients, or those who were tracheotomized during an acute decompensation episode.

Intermediate results on the first 58 patients included in the study (Raphael et al., 1992c) showed that the patients ventilating by nasal mask were the least severely affected at the moment of inclusion (Table 3). However, when survival as a function of the first technique of home ventilation used is analysed, it can be seen that deaths are more frequent in the NIPPV group than in those ventilated by tracheotomy (Fig. 1). Abdominal compression seems to be a potentially useful technique (Fig. 1), but it must be noted that this technique was only used in one of the 18 centres which participated in the multicentric study. A greater number of centres using this treatment and a larger number of participating patients will be necessary to evaluate this method of ventilation properly.

Table 2. Imperative ventilation and preventive ventilation in Duchenne's muscular dystrophy

			Mechanical ventilation techniques used and criteria for choice
Imperative ventilation		VC < 20 %	NIPPV, TIPPV or ACIPPV
	or	$PaCO_2 > 45$ mmHg	
	or	$PaO_2 < 60$ mmHg	
	or	2 episodes of respiratory insufficiency requiring endotracheal ventilation	Choice is made according to a decision-making scheme
	or	Patient ventilated for an acute episode who cannot be weaned from MV	In a patient who is already on NIPPV, this will be continued but the duration increased. In failure or contra-indication, TIPPV will be used
Preventive ventilation		Tracheotomy for any reason. 50 % > VC ≥ 20%. None of the criteria for necessary ventilation	NIPPV Randomized preventive trial Change to necessary ventilation, if any of the 6 criteria for necessary ventilation appear

Abbreviations: MV = mechanical ventilation; VC = vital capacity (% of predicted value); NIPPV = intermittent positive pressure ventilation by nasal mask; TIPPV = intermittent positive pressure ventilation by tracheotomy; ACIPPV = intermittent positive pressure ventilation by abdominal compression.

Table 3. Characteristics of patients receiving imperative ventilation (mean ± SD)

	NIPPV (n = 32)	TTIPV (n = 15)	ACIPPV (n = 11)
Age (years)	19 ± 5	21 ± 4	9 ± 3
PaO_2 * (mmHg)	76 ± 15	49 ± 26	60 ± 4
$PaCO_2$ * (mmHg)	46 ± 11	65 ± 17	50 ± 2
VC (ml)	735 ± 203	57 ± 73	846 ± 235
PaO_2 ** (mmHg)	93 ± 6	90 ± 10	81 ± 8
$PaCO_2$ ** (mmHg)	39 ± 5	33 ± 7	41 ± 4
Initial duration of ventilation per days (h)	8 ± 4	18 ± 6	12 ± 1

* During spontaneous breathing with $FiO_2 = 0.21$; ** During mechanical ventilation with $FiO_2 = 0.21$. For abbreviations, see Table 2.

It would be inappropriate to draw conclusions from these preliminary results. However, it seems that the nasal ventilation technique requires extremely rigorous surveillance in this evolutive disorder, which is not always easy to accomplish in the home setting. Participating members of the multicentric group have been informed of this result. The second intermediary analysis which covers 98 individuals (Raphael et al., 1992b) has shown that survival after 2 years is 61 per cent in the group using nasal ventilation and 70 per cent in the tracheotomy group. The difference in mortality between the two groups is less, but still persists.

This work has been complemented by a study of the quality of life which was carried out by psychologists in the homes of 28 patients (Andronikof-Sanglade et al., 1992). The intelligence

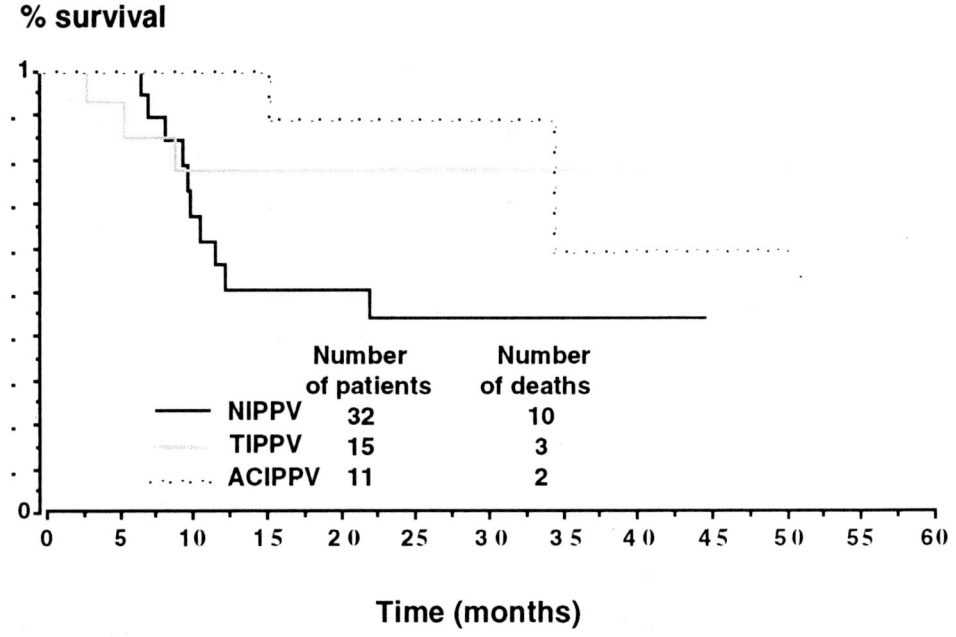

Fig. 1. Imperative ventilation. Survival according to initial method of ventilation.

quotient of these individuals is completely normal, and they enjoy a rich emotional life, but they suffer from social isolation and a lack of outlets for expressing their creativity. About half of them present signs of depression as indicated by the Rorschach test. Mechanical ventilation including tracheotomy is well tolerated. Nevertheless, the majority of patients questioned regretted that the physicians did not give them more information in advance on ventilation techniques, and on tracheotomy in particular.

An important point has also been noticed by others (Baydur *et al.*, 1990), that for an indication for imperative ventilation, nasal ventilation may be considered as a temporary measure which will sooner or later have to be replaced by tracheotomy. The medical question is to decide on the moment when this decision must be implemented.

A major effort in communication between physicians and patients is needed, in order to explain the advantages and drawbacks of the various techniques. More generally, when this study is complete, it might provide guidance in the choice of the mode of home ventilation in Duchenne's muscular dystrophy, in terms of both survival and quality of life.

Preventive ventilation

Preventive ventilation has a totally different objective from imperative ventilation. The question here is to discover whether early utilization of mechanical ventilation would delay the theoretically inevitable aggravation of the restrictive syndrome in patients who, at the beginning of ventilation, do not present any of the criteria for imperative ventilation. Theoretically, periodic hyperinsufflation of the pulmonary parenchyma could be beneficial. The decrease in force generated by the respiratory muscles is in fact accompanied by a decrease in pulmonary compliance which accelerates the reduction in vital capacity (Braun & Rochester, 1979), raises the respiratory workload, and undoubtedly favours fatigue of the respiratory muscles. The mechanism for the lowering of pulmonary compliance is not known with certainty, but it may be due to microatelectasia.

Periodic hyperinsufflation of the lung might prevent this phenomenon, as has been suggested for the respiratory sequelae of poliomyelitis (Ferris & Pollard, 1960). The decrease in parietal compliance due to kyphoscoliosis, retractions of the tendons, and costal deformations (Estenne et al., 1983) are other arguments in favour of the use of preventive ventilation. It has been shown, however, that hyperinsufflation for 15 min did not modify pulmonary compliance in the short term in ten patients with various neuromuscular diseases (de Troyer & Deisser, 1981).

In practice, intermittent positive pressure ventilation by mouthpiece is widely used in numerous pathologies. In 1982, in France, this was the method prescribed for 45 per cent of all 3120 patients with various disorders serviced by the regional associations for respiratory-insufficient individuals (Brambilla & Ludot, 1983). However, a therapeutic trial which included 985 patients with chronic obstructive bronchitis did not show a significant difference in survival between the control group and the group treated with intermittent positive pressure (Intermittent Positive Pressure Breathing Trial Group, 1983). IPPV was prescribed for 10 min, three times per day, but only 50 per cent of the patients adhered to this regimen which was none the less of short duration; the efficacy of positive intermittent pressure ventilation has therefore not been proven.

Nocturnal NIPPV is *a priori* a technique which is less constraining and better accepted than daily intermittent positive pressure ventilation by mouth. This technique was in fact first proposed for Duchenne's muscular dystrophy at an early stage, and later on extended to other neuromuscular disorders and to individuals presenting sleep apnoea. Sleep apnoea and nocturnal desaturations have been observed in Duchenne's muscular dystrophy at an early stage (Smith et al., 1987, 1988, 1989). This may favour the appearance of diurnal respiratory insufficiency as has been observed in other neuromuscular diseases (Bye et al., 1990). Nocturnal NIPPV which helps in these disorders might postpone the appearance of respiratory insufficiency by these mechanisms. This has been another argument in favour of early use of nasal mechanical ventilation in Duchenne's muscular dystrophy. However, there has been no demonstration in the literature of the efficacy of preventive NIPPV. Nasal mechanical ventilation is a technique which is constraining for the patient and its morbidity and cost are not negligible.

These then are the reasons which prompted us to organize a randomized trial with the purpose of evaluating the efficacy of nasal mechanical ventilation at an early stage in Duchenne's muscular dystrophy.

This trial involved patients who had none of the criteria for necessary ventilation (Table 2). If one of these criteria appeared during the study, imperative ventilation was prescribed immediately. The study compared the effect of 6 h nocturnal NIPPV with abstention. The end-point criterion was the appearance of hypercapnia of over 45 mmHg measured during spontaneous ventilation. The hypothesis used was that the median time for this level of hypercapnia to be reached would be 3 years in the control group and 5 years in the nasal mechanical ventilation group. For a risk of $\alpha = 0.10$ and $\beta = 0.10$, 125 patients were required for each group, or a total of 250 patients.

This study was begun in October 1986. The first intermediary analysis, provided for in the protocol and carried out on 62 patients (31 ventilated, 31 controls) on 1 June 1990, showed that the risk of death was increased in the nasal mechanical ventilation group (Raphael et al., 1990). This unexpected finding led us to halt enrolment of new patients into the study, in agreement with the Ethics Committee of the Société de Réanimation de Langue Française, and to use survival only as the end-point.

Definitive analysis carried out on 70 patients confirmed that the risk of death was higher in the ventilated group, and that the decrease in vital capacity was the same for the two groups (Raphael *et al.*, 1992a). These results were recently published (Raphael *et al.*, 1994). There are no arguments in favour of using preventive ventilation in Duchenne's muscular dystrophy.

In conclusion, it is to be hoped that this work will lead to better management of these patients, and an increase in their survival and quality of life. The strategy proposed here could be applied to other neuromuscular disorders of both children and adults. This type of study is the only means of convincing the public and physicians of the usefulness of these techniques.

References

Alexander, M.A., Johnson, E.W., Petty, J. & Stauch, D. (1979): Mechanical ventilation of patients with late stage Duchenne muscular dystrophy management in the home. *Arch. Phys. Med. Rehabil.* **60**, 289–292.

Andronikof-Sanglade, A., Benony, H., Montoux, F. & Raphael, J.C. (1992): Quelle qualité de vie pour des patients myopathes Duchenne de Boulogne ventilés à domicile? Société de Réanimation de Langue Française, Paris, 14–16 Janvier 1993. *Réan. Urg.* **1**, 1048 (abstract).

Bach, J.R., Alba, A.S., Bohatiuk, G., Saporito, L. & Lee, M. (1987a): Mouth intermittent positive pressure ventilation in the management of postpolio respiratory insufficiency. *Chest* **91**, 859–864.

Bach, J.R., O'Brien, J., Krotenberg, R. & Alba, A.S. (1987b): Management of end stage respiratory failure in Duchenne muscular dystrophy. *Muscle Nerve* **10**, 177–182.

Bach, J.R. & Alba, A. (1990): Management of chronic alveolar hypoventilation by nasal ventilation. *Chest* **97**, 52–57.

Bach, J.R., Campagnolo, D.I. & Hoeman, S. (1991): Life satisfaction of individuals with Duchenne muscular dystrophy using long-term mechanical ventilatory support. *Am. J. Phys. Med. Rehabil.* **70**, 129–135.

Baydur, A., Gilgoff, I., Prentice, W., Carlson, M. & Fischer, D.A. (1990): Decline in respiratory function and experience with long-term assisted ventilation in advanced Duchenne's muscular dystrophy. *Chest* **97**, 884–889.

Brambilla, C. & Ludot, A. (1983): Aspects socio-démographiques de l'insuffisance respiratoire chronique en France. *Rev. Fr. Mal. Resp.* **11**, 509–521.

Braun, N.M.Y. & Rochester, D.F. (1979): Muscular weakness and respiratory failure. *Am. Rev. Respir. Dis.* **119**, 123–125.

Bye, P.P., Ellis, E.R., Issa, F.G., Donnelly, P.M. & Sullivan, C.E. (1990): Respiratory failure and sleep in neuromuscular disease. *Thorax* **45**, 241–247.

Carroll, N. & Branthwaite, M.A. (1988): Control of nocturnal hypoventilation by nasal intermittent positive pressure ventilation. *Thorax* **43**, 349–353.

Colbert, A.P. & Schock, N.C. (1985): Respirator use in progressive neuromuscular diseases. *Arch. Phys. Med. Rehabil.* **66**, 760–762.

Curran, F.J. & Colbert, A.P. (1989): Ventilator management in Duchenne muscular dystrophy and postpoliomyelitis syndrome: twelve years' experience. *Arch. Phys. Med. Rehabil.* **70**, 180–185.

Delaubier, A., Guillou, C., Mordelet, M. & Rideau, Y. (1987): Assistance ventilatoire précoce par voie nasale dans la dystrophie musculaire de Duchenne. *Agressologie* **28**, 737–738.

de Troyer, A. & Deisser, P. (1981): The effects of intermittent positive pressure breathing on patients with respiratory muscle weakness. *Am. Rev. Respir. Dis.* **124**, 132–137.

Ellis, E.R., Bye, P.T.P., Bruderer, J.W. & Sullivan, C.E. (1987): Treatment of respiratory failure during sleep in patients with neuromuscular disease. Positive-pressure ventilation through a nose mask. *Am. Rev. Respir. Dis.* **135**, 148–152.

Estenne, M., Heilporn, A., Delhez, L., Yernault, J.C. & de Troyer, A. (1983): Chest wall stiffness in patients with chronic respiratory muscle weakness. *Am. Rev. Respir. Dis.* **128**, 1002–1007.

Ferris, B.G. & Pollard, D.S. (1960): Effect of deep and quiet breathing on pulmonary compliance in man. *J. Clin. Invest.* **39**, 143–149.

Gilgoff, I., Prentice, W. & Baydur, A. (1989): Patient and family participation in the management of respiratory failure in Duchenne's muscular dystrophy. *Chest* **95**, 519–524.

Granata, C., Capelli, T., Schiavina, M., Fabiani, A., Ballestrazzi, A., Sabattini, L., Corbascio, M. & Merlini, L. (1989): Ventilation mécanique dans la dystrophie musculaire de Duchenne de Boulogne. *Sem. Hop. Paris* **65**, 1037–1041.

Heckmatt, J.Z. (1987): Respiratory care in muscular dystrophy. *Br. Med. J.* **295**, 1014.

Heckmatt, J.Z., Loh, L. & Dubowitz, V. (1990): Night-time nasal ventilation in neuromuscular disease. *Lancet* **335**, 579–582.

Inkley, S.R., Oldenburg, F.C. & Vignos, P.J. (1974): Pulmonary function in Duchenne muscular dystrophy related to stage of disease. *Am. J. Med.* **56**, 297–306.

Intermittent Positive Pressure Breathing Trial Group (1983): Intermittent positive pressure breathing therapy of chronic obstructive pulmonary disease: a clinical trial. *Ann. Intern. Med.* **99**, 612–620.

Kerby, G.R., Mayer, L.S. & Pingleton, S.K. (1987): Nocturnal positive pressure ventilation via nasal mask. *Am. Rev. Respir. Dis.* **135**, 738–740.

Leger, P., Jennequin, J., Gerard, M. & Robert, D. (1989): Home positive pressure ventilation via nasal mask for patients with neuromusculoskeletal weakness or restrictive lung or chest-wall disease. *Respir. Care* **34**, 73–77.

Miller, J.R., Colbert, A.P. & Schock, N.C. (1988): Ventilator use in progressive neuromuscular disease: impact on patients and their families. *Dev. Med. Child. Neurol.* **30**, 200–207.

Mohr, C.H. & Hill, N.S. (1990): Long-term follow-up of nocturnal ventilatory assistance in patients with respiratory failure due to Duchenne-type muscular dystrophy. *Chest* **97**, 91–96.

Raphael, J.C., Chastang, C.L., Robert, D., Reybet-Degat, O., Charpak, Y., Muir, J.F., Gajdos, P.H., Cardinaud, J.P., Steenhouwer, F., Wattel, F. & Duroux, P. (1986): Assistance à domicile des handicapés respiratoires graves. Etude de la concordance des décisions thérapeutiques. Premier Colloque CNAMTS-INSERM "De la recherche biomédicale à la pratique des soins", Paris, 26–27 November 1985. *Editions INSERM* **144**, 577–586.

Raphael, J.C. (1987): Ventilation mécanique à domicile dans la dystrophie musculaire de Duchenne de Boulogne. Ventilation de nécessité et ventilation de prévention. Editorial. *Rev. Mal. Resp.* **4**, 195–197.

Raphael, J.C., Gajdos, P.H. & de Lattre, J. (1987): Handicap respiratoire chronique d'origine neuromusculaire. Physiopathologie. Perspectives thérapeutiques. In: *Fonction diaphragmatique, Travail respiratoire*, Limoges, 21–23 May 1987. Monographie de la Société de Réanimation de Langue Française, pp. 203–228. Paris: Expansion Scientifique.

Raphael, J.C., Chevret, S., Chastang, C.L., Bouvet, F. & le Groupe Multicentrique sur l'Evaluation de la Ventilation Mécanique à Domicile dans la DMDB (1990): Evaluation de la ventilation nasale de prévention dans la dystrophie musculaire de Duchenne de Boulogne (DMDB). Résultats intermédiaires d'une étude randomisée. Société de Réanimation de Langue Française, Paris, 22–25 November 1990. *Réan. Soins Intens. Méd. Urg.* **6**, 517 (abstract).

Raphael, J.C., Chevret, S., Chastang, C.L., Bouvet, F. & le Groupe Multicentrique sur l'Evaluation de la Ventilation Mécanique à Domicile dans la DMDB (1992a): Evaluation de la ventilation nasale de prévention dans la dystrophie musculaire de Duchenne de Boulogne (DMDB). Société de Réanimation de Langue Française, Paris, 16–18 January 1992. *Réan. Urg.* **1**, 121 (abstract).

Raphael, J.C., Chevret, S., Chastang, C.L., Bouvet, F. & le Groupe Multicentrique sur l'Evaluation de la Ventilation Mécanique à Domicile dans la DMDB (1992b): Evaluation des différents moyens de ventilation mécanique à domicile (VAD) dans la dystrophie musculaire de Duchenne de Boulogne (DMDB). Résultats intermédiaires d'une étude prospective multicentrique. Société de Réanimation de Langue Française, Paris, 14–16 January 1993. *Réan Urg*, **1**, 1034 (abstract).

Raphael, J.C., Chevret, S., Chastang, C.L., Bouvet, F. & the French Multicentric Group. (1992c): A prospective multicentre study of home mechanical ventilation in Duchenne de Boulogne muscular dystrophy. *Eur. Respir. Rev.* **2**, 312–316.

Raphael, J.C., Chevret, S., Chastang, C.L., Bouvet, F. & the French Multicenter Cooperative Group on Home Mechanical Ventilation Assistance in Duchenne de Boulogne Muscular Dystrophy (1994): Randomised trial of preventive nasal ventilation in Duchenne muscular dystrophy. *Lancet* **343**, 1600–1604.

Rideau, Y. (1986): The Duchenne muscular dystrophy child. Care of wheelchair-dependent patient. Death prevention. VIe International Congress on Neuromuscular Diseases. *Muscle Nerve* **9**, 55 (abstract)

Rideau, Y. (1987): Acharnement contre une maladie incurable, la dystrophie musculaire de Duchenne. *Agressologie* **28**, 733–735.

Rideau, Y. & Delaubier, A. (1988): Management of respiratory neuromuscular weakness. *Muscle Nerve* **11**, 407–408.

Segall, D. (1988): Noninvasive nasal mask-assisted ventilation in respiratory failure of Duchenne muscular dystrophy. *Chest* **93**, 1298–1300.

Smith, P.E.M., Calverley, P.M.A., Edwards, R.H.T., Evans, G.A. & Campbell, E.J.M. (1987): Practical problems in the respiratory care of patients with muscular dystrophy. *N. Engl. J. Med.* **316**, 1197–1205.

Smith, P.E.M., Calverley, P.M.A. & Edwards, R.H.T. (1988): Hypoxemia during sleep in Duchenne muscular dystrophy. *Am. Rev. Respir. Dis.* **137**, 884–888.

Smith, P.E.M., Edwards, R.H.T. & Calverley, P.M.A. (1989): Ventilation and breathing pattern during sleep in Duchenne muscular dystrophy. *Chest* **96,** 1346–1351.

Chapter 14

Genetic counselling in neuromuscular disorders

Gian Antonio Danieli and Maria Luisa Mostacciuolo

Department of Biology, University of Padua, Via Trieste 75, 35121 Padua, Italy

Summary

Genetic couselling is a communication process between the counsellor and the proband, dealing with the genetic implications of a given disease. After a diagnosis is established, the genetic risk can be estimated precisely, provided that all available information about the family is disclosed. Therefore, fiduciary relationships between proband and counsellor, based on informed consent, are the prerequisite for successful genetic counselling.

The counsellor is positively bound to secrecy about the family information. He is also obliged to act 'in favour' of the proband, while respecting his autonomy. In no instance can genetic counselling be directive. The counsellor's duty is to inform the proband about the nature of the disease, the pattern of inheritance, the risk of transmission in a given union, and the available options for preventing the occurrence of an unwanted pregnancy or for avoiding the birth of an affected child. The safety and efficacy of genetic tests must be clearly explained and the quality of the proband's understanding should be carefully evaluated.

The possibility of direct or indirect diagnosis of pathological mutations at the DNA level offers an unprecedented opportunity of success to the counsellor. However new problems have emerged, like the ethical and legal implications of pre-symptomatic DNA diagnosis. Some problems in genetic counselling of inherited neuromuscular disorders are briefly outlined.

The description of mendelian inheritance of some pathological conditions dates back to the beginning of this century (Garrod, 1902; Bateson, 1913). Since then, medical practice has exploited the family tree as a tool for predicting the possible occurrence of patients affected with a given genetic disorder. However, for at least 40 years the application of genetics to medicine was strongly conditioned by eugenics. The general attitude was in favour of the eradication of 'bad genes' in order to ameliorate the human breed, no matter if this eradication might have implied violence against people. Forced sterilization was massively applied in the USA and in Germany in the first decades of this century against feeble-minded persons, sexual offenders and people guilty of asocial behaviour. Later, under the Nazi government, euthanasia and mass killing became in Germany a state policy, in the name of eugenics ('*Rassenhygiene*') (Kevles, 1985). It was only after the end of the Second World War that horror at these crimes against mankind induced serious rethinking of eugenics. Almost at the same time, population genetics demonstrated the advantage of polymorphism in the evolutionary process (Dobzhanski, 1951; Lewontin, 1974). As a consequence, pathological traits were correctly interpreted as part of the natural genetic variability of the human species and a new trend emerged in genetic counselling – preventing the birth of newly affected cases is not a necessity for society, but a possibility for single persons or families to relieve their distress and anxiety. The benefit of the persons involved became the goal of counselling, which, in turn, hinged on the individual's right to be fully informed about genetic risk and on the right of a fully autonomous decision. At present, it is almost universally accepted that genetic counselling is a non-directive communication process to the proband, in order to give information about genetic risks and advice about the methods available to prevent the occurrence of new cases of the disease involved.

Genetic counselling cannot be prescribed; it must be offered by the doctor to the person affected with a genetic disease or to his/her relatives if they are worried about the possibility of giving birth to another affected person.

The doctor should explain to the proband what genetic counselling is and what are the possible outputs. The decision to be counselled should result from a sort of non-written informed consent, after a preliminary introductory talk.

Since the proband chooses to receive genetic counselling from a specific person, fiduciary relationships are automatically established between the proband and the counsellor. While the proband should feel the obligation to disclose all the available information about the family, the counsellor is positively obliged to secrecy about such information and to act 'in favour' of the proband, but respecting his or her autonomy. An obvious prerequisite for successful genetic counselling is a correct diagnosis. Fortunately, the progress of molecular genetics is continuously bringing new tools for this purpose, from DNA analysis to Western blots, immunohistochemistry and biochemical tests. In any case, the preliminary duty of the counsellor is to check that diagnosis was clearly established by reliable methods.

The second step is to estimate the risk of transmission of the genetic disease. For this purpose, after having reconstructed the family tree with the aid of the proband (and possibly of other members of the family), the risk of recurrence of a mendelian disease is easily computed by the aid of Bayesian logic (Stevenson & Davidson, 1976). The same method can also be applied to estimates of the recurrence risk for mendelian traits with reduced penetrance or for multifactorial diseases.

In several instances, DNA analysis can directly or indirectly (through the definition of the affected haplotype and linkage analysis) identify those individuals who are carrying the mutant (pathological) allele. This kind of approach implies that DNA samples can be obtained from all relevant members of the family. The doctor should be aware that blood sampling for DNA analysis can be prescribed only for diagnostic purposes for a person who is otherwise suspected to be affected. If this is not the case, a blood sample for DNA analysis can be obtained from relatives of an affected person only on a a voluntary basis. Each relative is free to refuse to give a blood sample for DNA analysis and equally free to refuse to know the result of the study. Paradoxically, the explanation of these individual rights to the members of the family may help in obtaining the DNA samples since, in the end, for each person involved the prevailing motivation will be to give 'help' to the proband, and the anxiety generated by knowing his own genotype may be temporarily removed by the possibility of postponing the problem in time.

Written informed consent should be given by each person from whom a blood sample is taken for DNA analysis. On the same form there should be a declaration, signed by the head of the laboratory, about the strict privacy of the genetic information and about the obligation of using such DNA only for purposes with which the person expressed his agreement.

Once the genetic risk is assessed (by Bayesian calculation or with the aid of DNA analysis or biochemical tests) the next problem is to communicate the risk to the proband. It is a general experience in genetic counselling that the simple communication to a proband that he/she is a carrier of a genetic disease which has occurred in the family induces a sense of guilt and strong anxiety (for him/herself or for the progeny).

Very often there is a wrong perception of the real risk (over-evaluation or under-evaluation), and hence an inadequate response to the situation is likely to follow. Therefore, a clear explanation of the 'real risk', in comparison with the standard risk of the general population, should be always provided to the proband.

After having clarified this point, the available options for preventing unwanted pregnancies or for avoiding the birth of an unwanted affected child should be clearly illustrated and discussed.

For those choosing to accept an at-risk pregnancy, the safety and efficacy of genetic tests must be clearly explained and the quality of the proband's understanding should be carefully evaluated.

In particular, the understanding of 'prenatal diagnosis' must be ascertained; in some cases an early prenatal diagnosis may be accepted because the woman believes that early therapy is possible. The later discovery of the true position may cause sorrow and anguish. The possibility of direct or indirect diagnosis of pathological mutations at DNA level offers to the counsellor an unprecedented opportunity of success. However, new problems have emerged, such as the ethical and legal implications of pre-symptomatic DNA diagnosis.

Frequently, DNA analysis is extended to the highest possible number of family members, in order to obtain more precise linkage information. This approach is ethically acceptable only if each subject is fully informed about the possible output of the analysis. Actually, two different kinds of results are expected from the study: not only a better definition of the genetic condition of the proband (or of the index case), but also of the genetic condition of the involved subject. Hypothetically, he might willingly participate in the study for the sake of the proband, but he might not be interested in being diagnosed. Moreover, the subject might be strongly against the idea of obtaining a pre-symptomatic 'DNA diagnosis' if the information on the condition might be adversely used by insurance companies or by managers. More generally, it is doubtful that an early pre-symptomatic 'DNA diagnosis' of incurable late-onset diseases might be somehow helpful for the involved person.

In any case, when different relatives of an affected family are involved, the result of the DNA analysis (and the communication of the genetic risk) should be given individually and separately to each subject, in order to preserve the privacy of the genetic information.

The problem is even more complicated when dealing with 'DNA diagnosis' in children. Obviously, the authorization for blood sampling and DNA analysis requires the informed consent of the parents. However, the parents' right to know the genotype of their sons and daughters is restricted to those diseases which are manifested in childhood or early adulthood, i.e. at the time in which parents are fully responsible for their progeny. Although parents may be strongly emotionally involved in facts concerning their children, it is hard to admit that they have a real right to extend their 'protection' beyond the onset of adulthood.

However, it may happen that the linkage study in a family with a late-onset genetic disease requires DNA typing of a child: in this case the parents should be asked to give consent for the blood sampling, in order to facilitate the definition of the proband's genetic risk, but they should be warned that they will not receive information about the results of the study.

This attitude may appear rather cruel, but it is gaining acceptance among genetic counsellors, since it is believed that the quality of life of the involved children would be different in the presence of such information. One important issue in genetic counselling is to establish a long-term relationship with the proband. In any family the nature of the problems is likely to change over time; moreover, the speed of progress in molecular diagnosis and disease-gene mapping may give new clues to the definition of genetic risks.

In current genetic counselling practice, the proportion of cases for whom the situation does not require an update or a further evaluation is minimal. Therefore, the regular follow up of a proband's situation should become routine practice. However, this would represent a very great workload for the counsellor and it would imply, at the end, a limitation in the number of probands who might benefit from counselling between the counsellor and the specialist or the family doctor.

Ideally, each single case should be discussed with the doctor involved before the genetic risk is communicated to the proband. This is really difficult to do in practice, but it should always be attempted. A good minimal rule is to ask the proband for authorization to send the doctor a copy of the written report on the definition of the genetic risk. In this way the doctor may be encouraged to contact the counsellor for further information.

Table 1(A). Mode of inheritance and gene location of some hereditary neuromuscular disorders

	Muscular dystrophies		
Duchenne/Becker	X-linked recessive	*	Xp21.2
Duchenne-like	Autosomal recessive		13q12
	Autosomal recessive	*	17q12–q21.33
Emery–Dreyfuss	X-linked recessive		Xq28
Facioscapulohumeral	Autosomal dominant		4q35
	Autosomal dominant		?
Limb-girdle	Autosomal dominant		5q
	Autosomal recessive		15q
	Autosomal recessive		2p
	Congenital myopathies		
Central core disease	Autosomal dominant	*	19q13.1
Fukuyama	Autosomal recessive		9q31–q33
Merosin deficiency	Autosomal recessive	*	6q2
Myotubular myopathy	X-linked recessive		Xq28
Nemaline myopathy	Autosomal dominant		1q21–q23
	Myotonic syndromes and ion channel diseases		
Becker's disease	Autosomal recessive	*	7q35
Epis.ataxia/myokymia	Autosomal dominant	*	12p
Hyperkal.period.paral.	Autosomal dominant	*	17q13.1–q13.3
Hypokal. period. paral.	Autosomal dominant	*	1q31–q32
Malignant hyperthermia	Autosomal dominant	*	19q13.1
	Autosomal dominant		17q11.2–q24
	Autosomal dominant		?
Paramyotonia congenita	Autosomal dominant	*	17q13.1–q13.3
Steinert's disease	Autosomal dominant	*	9q13
Thomsen's disease	Autosomal dominant	*	7q35
	Metabolic myopathies		
CPT deficiency	Autosomal recessive		11p11–p13
Glycogenosis type III	Autosomal recessive		17q23
Glycogenosis type V	Autosomal recessive	*	11q13
Glycogenosis type VII	Autosomal recessive	*	1cenq32
Glycogenosis type IX	X-linked recessive	*	Xq13
Glycogenosis type X	Autosomal recessive	*	7p12–p13
Glycogenosis type XI	Autosomal recessive	*	11p15.4

* Gene product identified; ? genetic heterogeneity proved, but locus unidentified.

Chapter 14   Genetic counselling in neuromuscular disorders

In the last 5 years unprecedented progress has occurred in the molecular genetics of neuromuscular disorders and most of the corresponding loci have been mapped. For some diseases, the gene was identified and different mutations have been detected (Table 1). In spite of this apparent clarification, the possibility of genetic heterogeneity should always be taken into account by the counsellor, especially when dealing with rare diseases or with pathological conditions in which the locus was identified in a limited number of kindred.

Table 1(B). Mode of inheritance and gene location of some hereditary neuromuscular disorders

	Neurogenic syndromes		
ALS (familial)	Autosomal dominant	*	21q22
Friedreich's ataxia	Autosomal recessive		2q33–q35
Friedreich's ataxia	Autosomal recessive		9cen–q21
(with vit.E def.)	Autosomal recessive		8q
HMSN type Ia	Autosomal dominant	*	17p11.2
HMSN type Ib	Autosomal dominant	*	1q21–q23
HMSN type I	Autosomal dominant		?
HMSN type II	Autosomal dominant		1p35–p36
MSN type III	Autosomal dominant		1q21–q23
(Dejerine–Sottas)	Autosomal dominant		17p11.2
HMSN type IV	Autosomal recessive		8q
HMSN X-linked	X-linked dominant	*	Xq13
HMSN with no liability	Autosomal dominant	*	17p11.2
to pressure palsies			
Kennedy's disease	X-linked recessive	*	Xq21.–q22
Kugelberg–Welander	Autosomal recessive		5q11–q13
Machado–Joseph disease	Autosomal dominant		14q24.3–q32
Spinal cerebral atrophy	Autosomal dominant	*	6p23
Spinal cerebral atrophy	Autosomal dominant		12q23–q4.1
Spinal cerebral atrophy	Autosomal dominant		14q24.3–ter
	Autosomal dominant		?
Werdnig–Hoffman	Autosomal recessive		5q11–q13
	Hereditary paraplegias		
Spastic paraplegia	Autosomal recessive		8q
Spastic parapl. compl.	X-linked recessive		Xq27–q28
Spastic parapl. uncompl.	X-linked recessive	*	Xq21–q22
Strumpell disease	Autosomal dominant		2p
	Autosomal dominant		14q
	Other neuromuscular diseases		
Adrenoleucodystrophy	X-linked recessive		Xq28
Amyloid neuropathy	Autosomal dominant	*	18q11.2–q12.1
Amyloidosis type IV	Autosomal dominant	*	11q23–qter
Amyloidosis type V	Autosomal dominant	*	9q33
Cong. fibrosis of the			
extraocular muscles	Autosomal dominant		1 2cen
Dysautonomia (fam.)	Autosomal recessive		9q31–q33

For symbols see Table 1(A).

Genetic counselling in neuromuscular disorders mainly involves families with recurring cases of Duchenne's or Becker's muscular dystrophy, spinal muscular atrophies or myotonic dystrophy. Recent progress in DNA analysis and the successful application of early prenatal diagnoses are convincing an increasing number of people to contact genetic counselling services. While in the past the motivation was to avoid the birth of individuals carrying a very severe handicap (often lethal in early infancy or before adulthood), at present people are asking to avoid the birth of individuals affected with diseases which in some cases are compatible with life, reproduction and even a normal occupation.

There is an increasing demand for prenatal diagnoses for such conditions and this issue is likely to become the focus of scientific and ethical discussions in the next few years.

The problems currently encountered in genetic couselling for neuromuscular diseases are mostly linked to the difficulty of a clear differential diagnosis and to the communication of scientific information to the people involved. Additional problems include the difficulty of warning other family members about potential genetic risks of which they are completely unaware.

Counselling for Duchenne's and Becker's muscular dystrophy may be considered as a paradigm. In these diseases, although the clinical phenotype appears to be clearly recognizable, molecular evidence is always needed for genetic counselling purposes. For males with consistent clinical features, CK levels and muscle biopsy, immunohistochemistry and Western blot testing should be done first. If dystrophin is absent or reduced in amount or size, an alteration in the corresponding gene is expected and screening for mutations should be performed. At present, quick and cheap PCR methods are available to identify intragenic deletions and duplications. Semi-quantitative multiplex PCR can be applied as well to detect heterozygotes for such types of mutation (Saad *et al.*, 1993). Several point mutations can be detected by the current screening methods, like SSCP, HET or DSCA (Saad *et al.*, 1994). In general, the analysis should first look for those mutations which are reported frequently. The large number of exons of the dystrophin gene and the difficulties in detection makes the search for unknown point mutations expensive and time consuming.

Once a mutation in the dystrophin gene is identified in a patient with Duchenne's or Becker's muscular dystrophy, genetic counselling may appear to be relatively simple, since the mutation may be sought in carriers or in prenatal diagnosis. However, the occurrence of two different deletions in the same family has been reported in a limited number of families (Mostacciuolo *et al.*, 1994). Therefore, the screening for deletions, duplications and point mutations should be always very careful, even if the defect is already known. Moreover, one cannot be absolutely certain that in a given family the same clinical phenotype (e.g. Becker's muscular dystrophy) will recur in the following generation.

A difficulty exists in explaining to the involved persons that different mutations of the same gene may lead to a different clinical course and that in members of the same family the clinical presentation may differ. This problem is particularly relevant in another neuromuscular disease, myotonic dystrophy, where the anticipation phenomenon is related to the variation of the CTG amplification (Novelli *et al.*, 1993).

If the mutation in the dystrophin gene remains undetected, the haplotype study should be performed, taking into account the fact that the very high intragenic recombination rate (Grimm *et al.*, 1989) imposes the use of several polymorphic DNA markers along the entire gene. This is the present routine approach, after the patient's DNA has been screened for a number of already reported mutations.

It is well established that isolated cases of Duchenne's muscular dystrophy are more likely to derive from familial segregation (2/3) than from new mutation. DNA analysis is able to prove if an isolated case of Duchenne's muscular dystrophy is due to a new mutation. If this is the case, every pregnancy after the birth of the affected child should be considered 'at risk' because of the possibility of germinal mosaicism (Danieli & Barbujani, 1984; Wood & McGillivray, 1988; Barbujani *et al.*, 1990).

Screening for dystrophin mutations should also be proposed in cases with high CKaemia, myalgia, cramps, myoglobinuria and dilative cardiomyopathy, because several authors have reported dystrophin mutation in cases with apparently minimal skeletal muscle effects. Similarly, it should be proposed in cases with a provisional diagnosis of limb-girdle muscular dystrophy, since about 10 per cent of such diagnoses turned out to be in reality Becker's muscular dystrophy (Grimm *et al.*, 1989; Mostacciuolo *et al.*, 1993). It should always be remembered that a more severe clinical course might occur in another member of the same family in which a case with a mild effect was detected.

Once a molecular diagnosis is established and the mutation identified, the counsellor is frequently asked about the prognosis of the disease. In dystrophinopathies, usually, the 'reading frame rule' (Monaco *et al.*, 1988) allows the clinical course of the disease to be predicted, but several exceptions have been reported. The number of reports on a correlation between genotype and clinical phenotype is still too limited to allow general conclusions to be drawn. Therefore, the counsellor should be very cautious on this point.

Careful reconstruction of the family tree may reveal that other family branches are at risk of having received the mutant allele, although no affected cases have yet become apparent.

In this situation, if the counsellor directly contacts the at-risk subjects he definitely violates their privacy. On the other hand, he may feel somehow guilty if a new case should occur because of his decision to restrict his counselling only to the proband.

The counsellor is obliged to disclose to the proband all relevant facts and to act in his interest. Therefore, he should communicate to the proband that other members in the family are at risk ('relevant facts') and that, if a new case were to occur, the proband might be accused by his relatives of having concealed very important information. To avoid the possibility that the proband might be involved in a very difficult situation is precisely to act in the interest of the proband. The counsellor might help the proband in finding the best way to convince the at-risk subjects to contact him for further information.

The most difficult part of genetic counselling is discussion about the available options. Very often the counsellor is directly requested by the proband to say what he would do in his place. It is very difficult to explain to the proband that this is the only reply the counsellor cannot give, especially when the proband is clearly disoriented. The correct procedure to be followed is to explain again, in the clearest way, the pros and cons of each option. Eventually, it may be suggested to the proband to come back after some days, in order to discuss the problem again.

The participation of both partners in the genetic counselling session is very important, since decisions about reproduction involve both parents. The presence of a psychologist may be of great help in evaluating the size of the problem and the possible presence of a conflict between the partners.

Genetic counselling is a powerful tool in managing hereditary neuromuscular diseases, but its use is very limited in mitochondrial myopathies. In these cases no estimate of the recurrence risk is possible, except the prediction that sons and daughters of an affected female will receive the mutant mitochondria, while the descendants of an affected male will be free from risk. Due to the peculiar pattern of inheritance, it is impossible to predict the severity of the effect in individuals who received the mutated mitochondria.

Genetic counselling is a complex process, which requires not only precise and updated knowledge of medical and molecular genetics, but also an objective view, a deep understanding of people's problems and an aptitude for interpersonal communication. The consequence of genetic counselling may be a reduced incidence of new cases of genetic diseases, but its most important goal should be the accomplishment of the personal right to know the genetic risk and to decide consequently.

References

Barbujani, G., Russo, A., Danieli, G.A, Spiegler, A.W.J., Borkowska, J. & Hausmanova Petrusewicz, I. (1990): Segregation analysis of 1885 DMD families: significant departure from the expected proportion of sporadic cases. *Hum. Genet.* **84,** 522–560.

Bateson, W. (1913): *Mendel's principles of heredity*, Chapter XII. Cambridge: Cambridge University Press.

Danieli, G.A. & Barbujani G. (1984): Duchenne muscular dystrophy: frequency of sporadic cases. *Hum. Genet.* **67,** 252–256.

Dobzhanski, T. (1951): *Genetics and the origin of species*, 3rd edn. New York: Columbia University Press.

Garrod, A.E. (1902): The incidence of alkaptonuria: a study in chemical individuality. *Lancet.* **ii,** 1616–1620.

Grimm, T., Mueller, B., Dreier, M., Kind, E., Bettecken, T., Meng, G. & Mueller, C.R. (1989): Hot spot of recombination within DXS164 in the Duchenne muscular dystrophy gene. *Am. J. Hum. Genet.* **45,** 368–372.

Kevles, D.J. (1985): *In the name of eugenics. Genetics and the uses of human heredity.* New York: A. Knopf.

Lewontin, R.C. (1974): *The genetic basis of evolutionary change.* New York: Columbia University Press.

Mostacciuolo, M.L., Miorin, M., Pegoraro, E., Fanin, M., Schiavon, F., Vitiello, L., Saad, F.A., Angelini, C. & Danieli, G.A. (1993): Reappraisal of the incidence rate of Duchenne and Becker muscular dystrophies on the basis of molecular diagnosis. *Neuroepidemiology* **12,** 326–330.

Monaco, A.P., Bertelson, C.J., Liechti-Gallati, S., Moser, H. & Kunkel, L. (1988): An explanation for phenotypic differences between patients bearing partial deletions of DMD locus. *Genomics* **2,** 90–95.

Mostacciuolo, M.L., Miorin, M., Vitiello, L., Rampazzo, A., Fanin, M., Angelini, C. & Danieli, G.A. (1994): Occurrence of two different intragenic deletions in two male relatives affected with Duchenne muscular dystrophy. *Am. J. Med. Genet.* **50,** 84–86.

Novelli, G., Gennarelli, M., Menegazzo, E., Mostacciuolo, M.L., Pizzuti, A., Fattorini, C., Terrarolo, D., Tomelleri, G., Giacanelli, M., Danieli, G.A., Rizzuto, N., Caskey, C.T., Angelini, C. & Dallapiccola, B. (1993): (CTG) Triplet mutation and phenotype manifestations in myotonic dystrophy patients. *Bioch. Med. Metab. Biol.* **50,** 85–92.

Saad, F.A., Galvagni, F. & Danieli, G.A. (1993): Rapid detection of human dystrophin gene mutations by multiplex semi-quantitative PCR. *BAM* **3,** 229–231.

Saad, F.A., Vita, G., Toffolatti, L. & Danieli, G.A. (1994): A possible missense mutation detected in the dystrophin gene by double strand conformation analysis (DSCA). *Neuromusc. Disord.* **4,** 335–341.

Stevenson, A.C. & Davidson, B.C.C. (1976): *Genetic counselling*, 2nd edn. London.: Heinemann Medical.

Wood, S. & McGillivray, B.C. (1988): Germinal mosaicism in Duchenne muscular dystrophy. *Hum. Genet.* **78,** 282–284.

Chapter 15

Molecular prenatal diagnosis of neuromuscular disorders

Bruno Dallapiccola,[1,2] **Francesca Capon,**[1] **Massimo Gennarelli,**[1]
Isabella Torrente,[1] **Rita Mingarelli**[1,2] **and Giuseppe Novelli**[1]

[1]*Department of Public Health, Università Tor Vergata, Via Tor Vergata, 135 EdE Nord, 00133 Rome, Italy;*
[2]*Ospedale C.S.S., I.R.C.C.S., Viale Cappuccini, 71013 San Giovanni Rotondo (FG), Italy*

Summary

Despite the wide range of prenatal diagnostic protocols, the monitoring of pregnancies at risk for mendelian disorders is ideally performed on DNA of chorionic villi sampled at around 10 weeks. At present, about 100 neuromuscular diseases can be monitored using a molecular approach. Some of these diagnoses, especially those based on linkage analysis, are time consuming and require extended pedigree studies. For this reason, characterization of the family before the beginning of pregnancy is recommended. The prenatal diagnosis of spinal muscular atrophy (SMA) illustrates some of the problems encountered during these studies, including the occasional need for recovery of DNA traces of a deceased patient from Guthrie cards, frozen biopsy or microscopy glass-slides; genetic heterogeneity; high frequency of *de novo* gene deletions. Nevertheless, personal experience with 76 SMA prenatal diagnoses supports a high accuracy for foetal predictions. Myotonic dystrophy exemplifies another neuromuscular disorder where the continuum spectrum of clinical severity is related to the instability of a dynamic AGC triplet. The close correlation between size of expansion and clinical outcome can be used to predict age at onset and disease severity during prenatal diagnosis studies as illustrated by personal experience with 61 cases. Future development of the prenatal diagnosis of neuromuscular disorders is mainly dependent on advances in mapping and cloning of the disease genes. Another promising issue is the development of first trimester non-invasive sampling protocols, based on the recovery of foetal cells circulating in the mother or degenerating trophoblast cells shed onto the endocervix by the 6th week of gestation.

Nowadays prenatal diagnosis techniques are widely used for monitoring pregnancies at risk throughout the gestation. This is an interdisciplinary effort where instrumental approaches devised for tissue sampling concur with cytogenetic, biochemical and molecular methods to evaluate the well-being of the embryo and foetus. In addition to the first and second trimester prenatal diagnosis protocols, based on chorionic villi sampling (CVS) around the 10th week of gestation, amniotic fluid sampling at 14 to 16 weeks, and cordocentesis-based recovery of foetal blood at 18 weeks, preimplantation diagnosis (PD) has become an alternative option for couples with no less than a one in four risk. This technique is based on embryo testing before implantation, followed by replacement in the mother of only the normal embryos. Some different PD protocols have been developed, including analysis of blastocysts recovered from the uterus on the fifth day following ovulation and fertilization, by flushing the uterine cavity via the cervix (so-called uterine lavage), and analysis of *in vitro* fertilized (IVF) embryos. In general, at the eight-cell stage a hole is made in the zona pellucida from which a single blastomere is removed. Alternative methods include trophoectoderm biopsy of 30–50 cells, or unfertilized egg first polar body removal through a hole made in the zona by micromanipulation prior to fertilization *in vitro* (Monk, 1992).

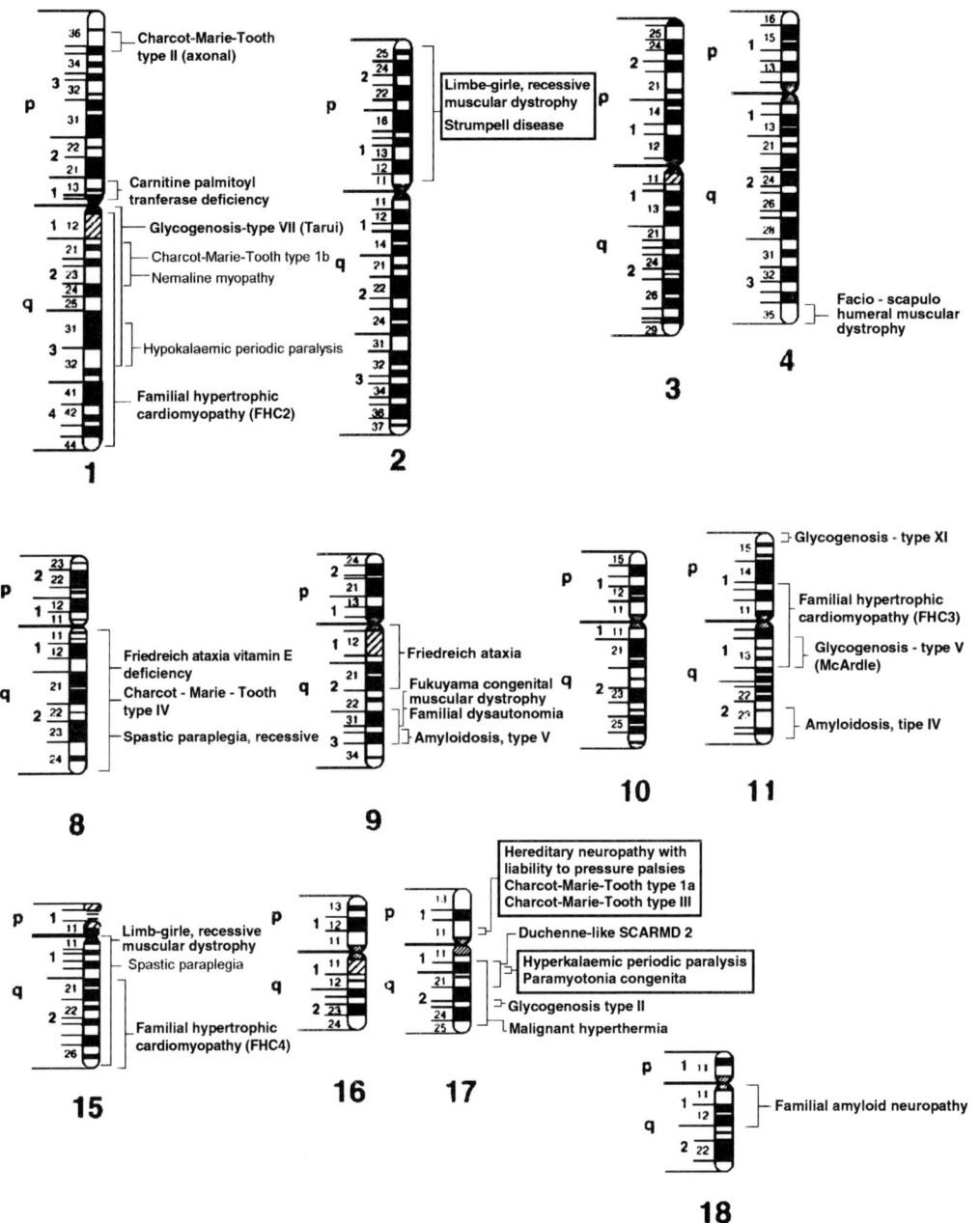

Fig. 1a. The human gene map of neuromuscular disorders, January 1995.

Chapter 15 Molecular prenatal diagnosis of neuromuscular disorders

Each of the tissue-sampling techniques has its own advantages and disadvantages (Table 1). However, the prenatal monitoring of pregnancies at risk for neuromuscular diseases, which is essentially based on foetal DNA analysis, is electively performed on trophoblast cells (CVS) recovered in the first trimester. At present PD, as well as other non-invasive methods of prenatal diagnosis, including

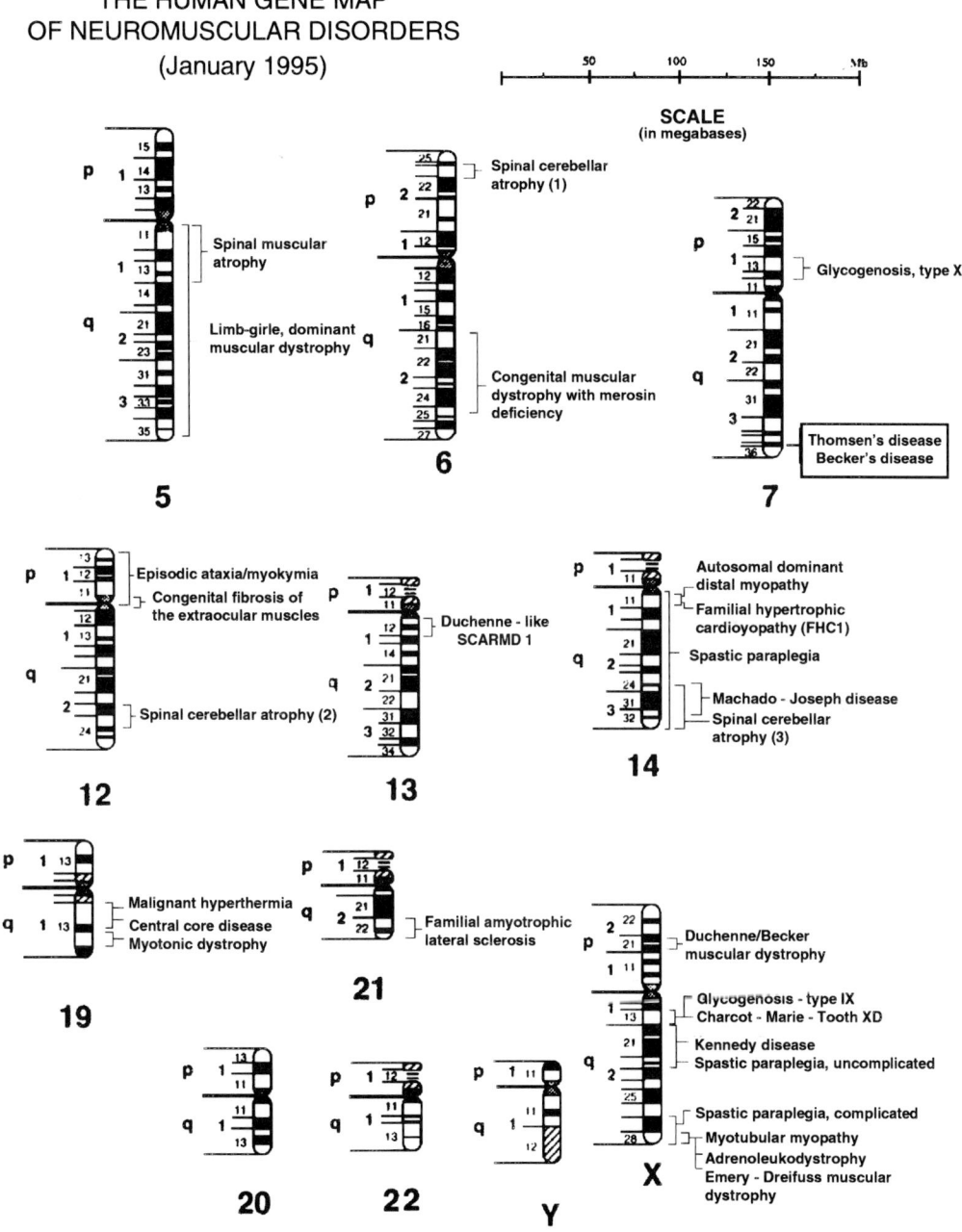

Fig. 1b. The human gene map of neuromuscular disorders, January 1995.

recovery of foetal lymphocytes, erythrocytes or syncytiotrophoblast elements from the maternal circulation (Adinolfi, 1992), or trophoblast cells in the cervical canal (Massari *et al.*, 1996) are only experimental and not yet amenable to large-scale application.

Table 1. Approaches to the prenatal diagnosis of genetic diseases

Parameters	PI	CVS	PAMN	AMN	FB	US
Time of diagnosis	E	E	E	L	L	L
Foetal risk	?	–	?	–	–	–
Test rapidity	++	++	–	–	++	+
Accuracy	+/–	+(CM)	+	+	+	–
Acceptability	–	+	+	+	–	+
Utilization	–	+	+/–	++	–	++
Cost/benefit	?	+	+	+	?	?
Other		Cost	DNA			

PI = preimplantation; CVS = chorionic villi sampling; PAMN = precocious amniocentesis; AMN = amniocentesis; FB = foetal blood; US = ultrasound; E = early; L = late; CM = chromosomal mosaicism.

The progress in foetal tissue sampling has been paralleled by striking advances in the mapping and cloning of human disease genes, which include over 60 genes related to neuromuscular disorders (Fig. 1) (Müller *et al.*, 1994; Kaplan & Fontaine, 1995). These advances have been favoured by dramatic changes in the methodology of gene searching.

In the past most genes were identified based on pre-existing knowledge of their biochemical defect. Although this strategy of 'functional cloning' was successful, biological information about the basic defect was available only for a limited number of disorders. This has accounted for the relatively slow progresses in human gene analysis. Mapping and cloning of human genes was revolutionized by the strategy of 'positional cloning', where mapping is essential to the process, and function is only determined after the gene has been isolated. This gene identification begins with collecting representative pedigrees in which the disease gene of interest is segregating. The family members are analysed with several polymorphic markers until one or more of them prove a linkage with the disease gene. This is shown by the consistent association of an allele with the disorder in a given family. For this purpose, mathematical methods are used, which predict the likelihood of positive linkage information. Fine mapping is also used for narrowing down the responsible region, by examining additional markers physically close to the marker which had shown a positive linkage. The 'candidate gene' approach is then used for testing if any of the genes previously assigned to the relevant region is related to the disease. The ultimate proof of the cloning of the disease gene is provided by sequence analysis and demonstration of mutations in the patients (Collins, 1992).

The medical consequences of gene identification are wide. DNA analysis corroborates clinical diagnosis, and improves understanding of genetic heterogeneity and genetic counselling. It also makes possible carrier-status testing in individual families, and the implementation of widespread population screening of common disease genes. It also allows presymptomatic testing of late-onset disorders and, most relevant to the present discussion, prenatal diagnosis.

An illustrative example is shown in Fig. 2, which refers to a pedigree in which the X-linked Charcot–Marie–Tooth (CMTX, MIM 302800) disease is segregating. When the mother at risk (subject III, 9) requested prenatal diagnosis in 1993, linkage analysis had assigned the disease gene to Xq13 (Gal *et al.*, 1985). DNA markers flanking the CMTX locus were analysed in the family to define the haplotype at risk, when the mother was in the first trimester of gestation. As is shown in the figure, the proband who had an *a priori* risk of one in two of carrying the mutation, was found to be homozygous for the wild-type genotype. Some practical issues arise from personal experience

Chapter 15   Molecular prenatal diagnosis of neuromuscular disorders

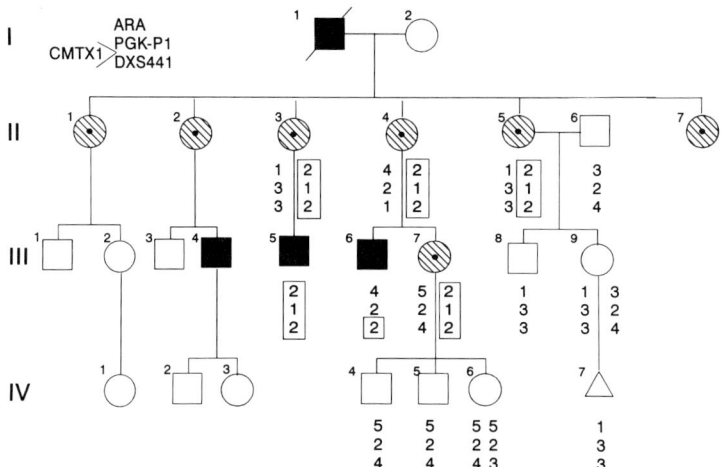

Fig. 2. Pedigree of a family with X-linked Charcot–Marie–Tooth disease. ARA, PGK-P1 and DXS441 markers flanking the disease gene in Xp13 have been used to identify the haplotype at risk which is shown in boxes.

with this family and have a general application for the molecular analysis of pregnancies at risk. First, proper genetic counselling should if possible be provided to these families before the beginning of pregnancy. This is in fact a unique opportunity for assessing the specific risk of any couple and planning the proper programme of prenatal monitoring. Second, molecular investigations of the relevant family members should be carried out before the beginning of pregnancy. In general, linkage studies are time consuming and occasionally cannot be concluded by the proper time when the foetus should be monitored. Third, the accuracy of prenatal diagnosis is consistently increased by the direct search for gene mutations. The reliabililty of linkage analysis is directly related to the physical distance on the chromosome between the disease gene and the flanking polymorphic markers used to define the haplotype at risk. Admittedly, part of the laborious efforts, including blood collection from pertinent family members and linkage analysis, that were needed in 1993 to reach a diagnosis in this family could be shortened today. In fact, cloning of the connexin, the CMTX disease gene (Bergoffen et al., 1993), allows direct analysis of the mutation.

The amazing development of clinical molecular genetics encourages storing DNA samples from affected individuals at risk of dying and, when appropriate, material from terminations of pregnancies. Thus a major activity of any genetic centre should be DNA banking according to issued guidelines (Yates et al., 1989). It should be remembered that any molecular approach to prenatal diagnosis can only be as good as the clinical diagnosis and family history. Therefore it is mandatory that clinicians and molecular geneticists work hand in hand. This issue is illustrated by our personal experience with the prenatal diagnosis of spinal muscular atrophies (SMAs), as shown in Table 2.

SMA I (Werdnig–Hoffmann disease, MIM 253300) is a severe autosomal recessive disorder in which the patient dies in general by the age of 18 months. Until January 1995, when the SMA gene was cloned from region 5q12–14 (Lefebvre et al., 1995; Roy et al., 1995), the prenatal diagnosis protocols of this disorder were based on linkage analysis using DNA markers, flanking the SMA locus (Lo Cicero et al., 1994).

A minimum prerequisite for linkage-based genetic prenatal diagnosis is the presence in the family of an affected sibling. Comparative analysis of parents and patient defines the haplotype at risk. However, this analysis is often prevented by the early death of the patient. For this reason, we have used the recovery of DNA traces of probands, using Guthrie spots collected at birth, frozen tissue sections, paraffin-embedded tissues and microscopy glass-slides (slide-PCR). We have developed an original protocol based on PCR amplification of DNA microsatellites tightly linked to the SMA locus, to obtain specific amplified products. This procedure was successful in a series of cases in which frozen tissues or slides had been stored for 1 to 20 years (Capon et al., 1993a) (Fig. 3a). We have also overcome some technical difficulties due to viscosity of the embedding media. In particular, we have developed a reproducible and sensitive protocol for PCR amplification of DNA from biopsy sections mounted with Spurr's mixture. This is a low-viscosity embedding medium widely used in electron microscopy, where it provides a high-quality and rapid tissue infiltration. The protocol, which is essentially based on block depolymerization using tetrahydrofuran, in our hands has provided successful PCR amplification of all tested specimens (Capon et al., 1993b).

Table 2. Personal experience with SMA prenatal diagnosis

	SMA I	SMA II	SMA III	TOTAL
Total pregnancies with 1 in 4 risk (microsatellite analysis)	56	8	2	76
Proband DNA source				
Guthrie cards	2	–	–	2
Microscopic glass slide	6	–	–	6
Frozen muscle biopsy	8	–	–	8
Umbilical cord	1	–	–	1
Blood	39	18	2	59
Results				
Affected	11	6	1	18
Carrier	26	8	1	35
Non-affected	19	4	–	23
Retrospective deletion analysis				
NAIP gene deletions	12/20	3/13	0/2	15/35
SMN gene deletions	20/20	13/13	1/2	34/35

We have experimented with an even more extreme application of DNA-amplification technology in the monitoring of a pregnancy at risk for SMA I. In the family examined the first affected baby was dead and a healthy daughter was alive. Some people in this region of southern Italy (Calabria) from which this family originated used to keep the umbilical cord of their newborns, because of the superstitious belief that it is a charm. When these parents requested prenatal diagnosis at the eighth week in their third pregnancy, the mummified umbilical cord was the only available biological remains of the dead baby. At that time, we did not know that the molecular analysis would have been complicated by an additional problem – the parents had stored two indistinguishable umbilical cords, one belonging to the affected baby and the other to the healthy daughter. Nevertheless, DNA analysis has elegantly solved this puzzle. We analysed a set of microsatellites in the amplified DNA recovered from the two umbilical cord remains, and compared them with those in the parents, healthy daughter, and trophoblast sampled at 10 weeks' gestation. On this basis, we predicted that the foetus was an SMA heterozygote (Fig. 3b). This diagnosis was confirmed at the birth of a healthy baby.

In conclusion, some different technical tips allow reliable retrospective genotyping of archival tissues. This step is preliminary to the prenatal diagnosis of those lethal diseases in which patients are no longer available for direct DNA typing.

Linkage analysis was used for monitoring pregnancies at risk soon after the assignment of the three major forms of SMA to chromosome 5 (Brzustowicz et al., 1990; Gilliam et al., 1990). The accuracy of prediction was estimated to be in the range of 80 to 99 per cent, based on the genetic

Chapter 15   Molecular prenatal diagnosis of neuromuscular disorders

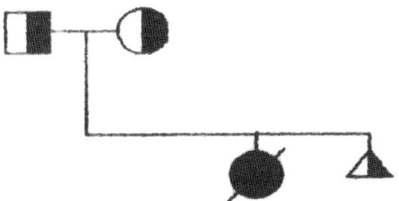

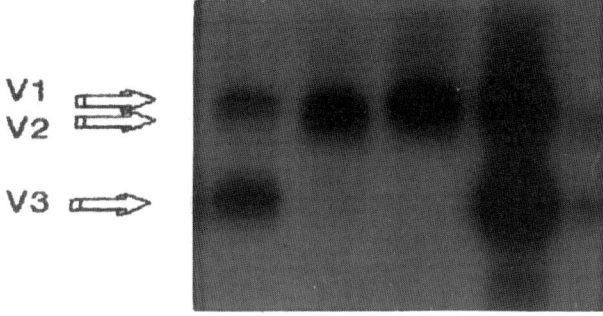

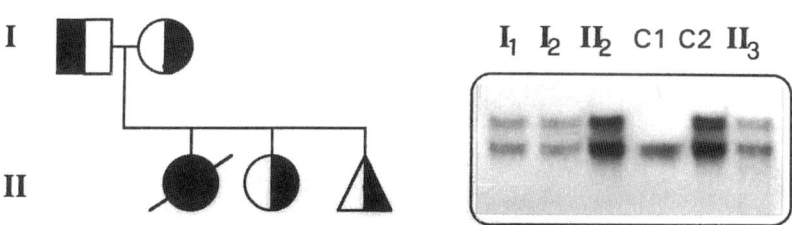

Fig. 3. Prenatal diagnosis in pregnancies at risk for SMA I. The haplotypes at risk have been assessed on DNA traces of the proband recovered from (a) microscopic glass slides; and (b) from mummified umbilical cord of the proband (C1) and her sister (C2).
In (a), the father is heterozygous for V1 and V3 alleles, the mother for V1 and V2. The affected deceased proband was heterozygous for the paternal V1 and maternal V2 alleles, which are the disease-associated alleles. The foetus at risk was heterozygous for the paternal V3-wild-type allele and for the V2 at-risk allele.
In (b), parents (I1 and I2), healthy daughter (II2) and one of the umbilical cords are similarly heterozygous for microsatellite markers. The second umbilical cord is homozygous for the low molecular weight allele, indicating the probable genotype of the deceased affected proband. The genotype found in the monitorized pregnancy (II3) is heterozygous as are the healthy relatives, suggesting that the foetus is heterozygous for SMA mutation.

distance between the markers and the disease locus (Daniels *et al.*, 1992; Lo Cicero *et al.*, 1994). Not less than 400 pregnancies at risk have been monitored in the world using segregation analysis of highly polymorphic markers. However, the occasional occurrence of a non-mendelian pattern of inheritance, including uniparental disomy, *de novo* deletions and genetic heterogeneity have consistently reduced the influence of linkage (Brzustowicz *et al.*, 1994; Capon *et al.*, 1996a; Novelli *et al.*, 1995a). Although uniparental isodisomy should be a rare event, it must be considered a possibility during prenatal diagnosis studies. *De novo* deletions were demonstrated in one or more subloci recognized by marker C212/C272 in 10 to 18 per cent of SMA I patients. These markers span several kilobases of the disease region and show linkage disequilibrium (non-random distribution of alleles around the disease gene).

The genetic heterogeneity of SMA has been documented in a limited number of families and represents a potential difficulty while providing prenatal diagnosis. It has been estimated that about 5 per cent of SMAs could not be linked to chromosome 5. Although the cloning of the SMA gene is expected to overcome this difficulty, personal experience with a prenatal diagnosis in a couple with a risk of one in four recommends caution in interpreting the results provided by linkage studies. The parents requesting the first trimester monitoring of their second pregnancy have had a daughter with a neonatal SMA I associated with early onset respiratory distress due to diaphragmatic paralysis. The diagnosis was supported by neurogenic muscular atrophy, a decrease in the motor neurones of the anterior horns of the spinal cord, degenerative changes and neuronophagia, and proliferation of astrocytes and microglia. This unique variant of SMA with early muscular involvement, weakness and atrophy of the distal musculature was considered a variant of the more classical SMA I (McWilliam *et al.*, 1985). Based on linkage analysis with five microsatellite markers flanking the SMA locus on 5q, we defined the parental 5q chromosomes segregated to the affected newborn and monitored the second pregnancy. The foetus was predicted to be unaffected, having inherited the parental haplotypes unlinked to the SMA locus on chromosome 5. At birth the baby presented with the same symptoms found in the first daughter and died 1 h after delivery. Molecular analysis of the newborn's DNA corroborated the CVS results. Having excluded misdiagnosis and non-paternity, we concluded that the SMA variant associated with paralysis of the diaphragm maps outside the critical 5q region, implying that this form is genetically different from classical SMA types (Novelli *et al.*, 1995b). This result has obvious implications for genetic counselling and prenatal diagnosis in SMA families.

The SMA region was characterized at the beginning of 1995 and two genes have been cloned, which are considered to be related to the disease – survival motor neuron (SMN), and neural apoptosis-inhibitory protein (NAIP) (Lefebvre *et al.*, 1995; Roy *et al.*, 1995). SMN is deleted in about 97–98 per cent of SMA patients, and NAIP in 45–58 per cent. This type of mutation, which is quite unusual in a mendelian disease, is related to the molecular complexity of this region, where multiple genes and pseudogenes are located encoding functional products and multiple transcripts (Pizzuti *et al.*, 1995). Two copies of SMN are found in normal chromosomes, namely SMNc and SMNt, each spanning 20 kb of genomic DNA. Only five single base pair substitutions distinguish the two forms and none of them seems critical to any function. Both copies of SMN are transcribed in lymphoblasts and muscle and show dosage effect in SMA patients (unpublished observation). Molecular analysis has demonstrated that only SMNt is deleted in the patients (Fig. 4a), while homozygous SMNc deletions do not have any obvious phenotypic effect. This behaviour complicates the direct molecular analysis of the disease, since only SSCP analysis distinguishes SMNt and SMNc. The complexity of the SMA locus suggests that SMN could be the SMA-determining gene, alone or in conjunction with NAIP (Fig. 4b) or other unknown genes. However, in the absence of a complete transcript and deletion breakpoint map, it is premature to speculate about the causative involvement of other genes in SMA. Present knowledge recommends caution in the prenatal testing of this disease, based on a single gene assay, although we and others have detected the 'SMA chromosomes' in all cases studied by direct gene testing (Lefebvre *et al.*, 1995; Capon *et al.*,

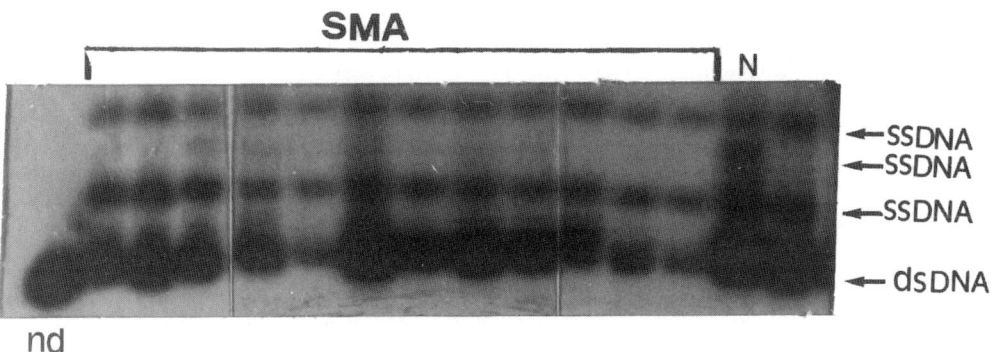

Fig. 4(a). Prenatal diagnosis of SMA I: (a) SSCP pattern of SMN exon 7 in SMA patients, compared to control (N).

1996b). Further studies are needed to define the molecular genetics of SMA and the feasibility of an accurate and reliable prenatal testing assay in families without a prior history of SMA or in which biological samples from an affected proband are impractical or not available.

During the past few years, we have acquired considerable experience on another neuromuscular disease, myotonic dystrophy (DM, MIM 160900), which also has relevance for prenatal diagnosis protocols. This autosomal dominant disorder is due to an unstable AGC triplet repeat. This mitotic and meiotic length variation (expansion) disrupts the kinetics of the DM gene transcription and the functioning of the gene product. The resulting multisystemic disease manifests with a quite variable clinical outcome. In fact, DM severity is a continuous spectrum, which varies from the late-onset to the most severe congenital cases (CDM), transmitted in general by affected mothers. The dynamics of the DM mutation are closely related to the phenotypic variability, larger expansion usually resulting into a more severe clinical involvement (Novelli et al., 1993a).

Analysis of the DM gene triplet has become a widely used method to support clinical diagnosis. In addition, the remarkable interfamilial and intrafamilial variability has made this molecular testing a useful approach for assessing age at onset, systems involved, anticipation and prognosis. Although

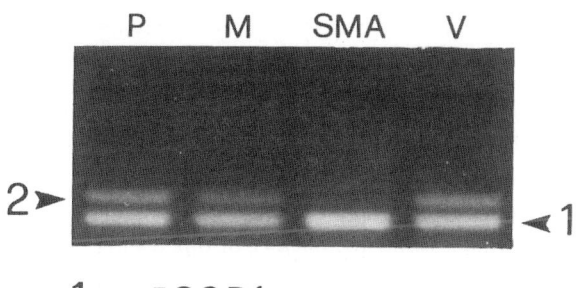

Fig. 4(b). The NAIP gene is deleted in the proband and undeleted in CVS, predicting unaffected foetus.
P = father; M = mother; SMA = affected proband;
V = chorionic villus.

genotype and phenotype at times do not match perfectly, in general the unstable mutation provides a biological basis to the broad range of clinical severity. This has been nicely shown by studies which have compared triplet expansions with age at onset, and clinical parameters. Although the strongest correlation was apparent betweeen the AGC amplification and muscle involvement, other clinical manifestations have also proved a definite relationship with the expansion (Novelli et al., 1993a; Mastrogiacomo et al., 1994; Melacini et al., 1995).

On the basis of triplet number, clinical outcome and age at onset, the DM patients have been divided into four classes. The mildest form, which occurs in middle to old age (late adult), is associated with 50 to a few hundred AGC; the classical adult-type, with myotonia and muscle weakness, has a few hundred to 1000 triplets; the juvenile form is due to many hundred to thousands of AGC; the congenital form shows thousands of triplets (Novelli et al., 1993b). However, the distribution of repeat lengths associated with the different clinical forms are wide and overlapping, and even within the same family similar triplet expansions are associated with discordant clinical outcomes (Novelli et al., 1993a). It is likely that at least part of this variability is related to somatic mosaicism. Another possibility is that this dynamic mutation causes an abnormal transcription of other *cis*-contiguous genes.

With the above limitations in mind, prenatal diagnosis has been offered to parents with a one in two risk of DM.

Prenatal diagnosis has become available on an experimental basis since 1983 using polymorphisms flanking the disease gene to trace the segregation of the DM chromosome. However, this approach provided no understanding of the molecular basis of intrafamilial clinical variability, and at the time results were not conclusive due to the impossibility of reconstructing the haplotype of deceased affected probands, family non-compliance, non-paternity and apparent crossover. Direct DNA-based diagnosis identifies individuals with the mutation, either symptomatic or not, carrying a *protomutation*, but 'at-risk' of expanding the [AGC] number at meiosis. Direct testing predicts the severity of the molecular changes in a way that can become a prognostic parameter. By re-examining the molecular status and clinical course of 468 DM patients, we developed a predictive molecular test based on the number of [AGC] triplets. According to the duration and severity of the disease, three different phenotypic classes have been recognized which match nicely with a normal distribution in three classes of [AGC] triplets. A statistical elaboration of data was performed to implement a predictive value of the clinical status by simply examining the genomic [AGC] number (Gennarelli et al., 1996). This has allowed us to carry out a retrospective analysis of 61 first trimester prenatal diagnoses monitored in Italy and in Spain (in collaboration with M. Baiget, Barcelona). Twenty-four foetuses were predicted to be affected having an [AGC] expansion in the range of 70 to 3100 triplets (Table 3). Seven foetuses fell in the range where the expected outcome is CDM (> 1500 AGC). Seven foetuses were considered to be at low risk for CDM (< 600 AGC). The other foetuses were predicted to develop an intermediate or severe form (range 600–1500 AGC). In all cases, parents elected for termination of pregnancy. All foetuses predicted to be unaffected were confirmed at birth by expansion analysis on blood DNA.

Personal experience has shown that accurate monitoring of at-risk pregnancies is possible and of great help in DM families. Nevertheless, the complexity of this testing recommends that the large scale implementation of this analysis is validated by the results of pilot projects and the achievement of appropriate levels of support and guidelines.

There is an increasing demand for those who provide prenatal diagnostic services to reduce the time taken to provide a diagnosis, and to develop reliable methods for testing earlier in pregnancy, widening the spectrum of available diagnoses, and reducing the invasiveness of foetal-cell sampling techniques. Much of this progress is related to advances in the mapping and cloning of disease genes and setting up of rapid strategies for their analysis. The map position has been defined for about 100 neuromuscular disorders, in half of which the gene has been also cloned. This has

Chapter 15   Molecular prenatal diagnosis of neuromuscular disorders

substantiated the splitting or lumping of individual diseases, and improved the genetic counselling elegibility.

Table 3. Personal experience on prenatal diagnosis in myotonic dystrophy

CVS	Parent	Δ
70	65 (M)	
80	80 (M)	–
200	200 (F)	–
300	300 (F)	–
350	350 (F)	–
500	400 (F)	100
600	300 (M)	300
670	500 (F)	170
800	300 (M)	500
900	180 (F)	720
1000	600 (M)	400
1200	200 (M)	1000
1200	200 (M)	1000
1200	1000 (M)	200
1250	700 (M)	550
1300	500 (M)	800
1300	500 (M)	800
1500	250 (M)	1250
1600	500 (M)	1100
1600	200 (M)	1400
1700	350 (M)	1350
1700	850 (M)	850
1800	750 (M)	1050
3100	800 (M)	2300

Results of AGC triplet expansions in 24 affected foetuses (CVS) compared to the expansion in the affected parent. M = mother; F = father. The difference (Δ) between the affected parent and foetus is also shown.

Among the development of non-invasive methods of foetal sampling, a topic of great interest and active research is the recovery of foetal nucleated cells, whether lymphocytes, erythrocytes or syncytiotrophoblastic elements present in the maternal circulation in very small numbers. Although it has been proved that prenatal diagnosis of selected inherited disorders can be achieved using this approach, the technique is still fraught with severe difficulties. One problem is to lyse the maternal contaminating cells, which is done with specific antibodies but is rarely complete. In addition, maternal immune responses may lyse foetal lymphocytes or erythrocytes expressing incompatible HLA or ABO antigens. Thus, the most promising cellular elements are syncytiotrophoblasts, although additional longitudinal investigations are needed before entering into routine testing. One major problem related to the use of these foetal cells for prenatal diagnosis purposes is that they cross the placenta only relatively late in gestation, when other invasive, but low-risk methods, are successfully available (Adinolfi, 1992).

An alternative method of non-invasive first trimester prenatal diagnosis is based on retrieval of trophoblast cells from the lower part of the uterine cavity. This approach could be effective after the sixth week of gestation, when the degenerating trophoblast sheds into the endocervix. These foetal cells can be collected for genetic analysis, by flushing the mucus from the canal, using physiological solution (Chasouat et al., 1994; Ishai et al., 1994; Pertl et al., 1994). Only a few studies have supported the effectiveness of this procedure in the molecular prenatal diagnosis of human diseases (Adinolfi et al.,1993; Bernini et al., 1994; Massari et al., 1996). In particular our group has recovered foetal DNA in slightly fewer than half of the transcervical cell samples recovered by endocervical canal flushing between weeks 7 and 9 of gestation. The sex predicted was confirmed in all foetuses by karyotype analysis of chorionic villi at 10 weeks. In addition the foetal genotype was correctly predicted in pregnancies at risk for spinal muscular atrophy, myotonic dystrophy, cystic fibrosis and thalassaemia, as shown by subsequent results on chorionic villi or newborns' leukocytes.

In conclusion, it appears that the transcervical retrieval of trophoblastic cells is a promising non-invasive technique for early prenatal molecular diagnosis of mendelian disorders. Several problems require to be overcome before the use of this method is recommended. They include improving the rate of foetal DNA recovery, evaluating the non-invasiveness of this sampling procedure by long-term follow up of the pregnancies, and reducing maternal contamination. At the molecular level, parental genotyping is required and it becomes mandatory when the mother is the affected parent or shares with her partner the same heterozygous disease-associated mutation.

Acknowledgments

This work was supported in part by Telethon, Italy (Grants n.511, 296 and 689), CNR, P.F. Ingegneria Genetica and Ministry of Health, Italy.

References

Adinolfi, M.C. (1992): Fetal nucleated cells in the maternal circulation. In: *Prenatal diagnosis and screening,* eds. D.J.H. Brock, C.H. Rodeck & M.A. Ferguson-Smith, pp. 651–660. London: Churchill Livingstone.

Adinolfi, M., Davies, A., Sharif, S., Soothill, P. & Rodeck, C. (1993): Detection of trisomy 18 and Y-derived sequences in fetal nucleated cells obtained by transcervical flushing. *Lancet* **342,** 231–233.

Bergoffen, J., Scherer, S.S. & Wang, S. (1993): Connexin mutations in X-linked Charcot–Marie–Tooth disease. *Science* **262,** 2039–2041.

Bernini, L.F., Kanhai, H.H.H., Losekoot, M., Giordano, P. & Harteveld, C.L. (1994): Prenatal diagnosis of homozygous α°-thalassemia by an immunological method. In: *Fetal cells in maternal blood,* eds. J.L. Simpson & S. Elias. *Ann. N. Y Acad. Sci.* **731,** 193–196.

Brzustowicz, L.M., Lehner, T., Castilla, L.H. *et al.* (1990): Genetic mapping of chronic childhood-onset spinal muscular atrophy to chromosome 5q11.2–13.3. *Nature* **344,** 540–541.

Brzustowicz, L.M., Allitto B.A., Matseoane, D., Theve, R., Michaud, L., Chatkupt, S., Sugarman, E., Penchaszadeh, G.K., Suslak, L., Kpenigsberger, M.R., Gilliam, T.C. & Handelin B.L. (1994): Paternal isodisomy for chromosome 5 in a child with spinal muscular atrophy. *Am. J. Hum. Genet.* **54,** 482–488.

Capon F., Melchionda, S., Gennarelli, M., Lo Cicero, S., Giacanelli, M., Novelli, G. & Dallapiccola, B.(1993a): A tool for the molecular analysis of an early lethal disease: slide-PCR in spinal muscular atrophy patients. *Mol. Cell Probe***7,** 221–226.

Capon, F., Lo Cicero, S., Novelli, G. & Dallapiccola B. (1993b): PCR protocol for DNA recovery from Spurr's-embedded muscle biopsies. *PCR Meth. Appl.* **3,** 211–212.

Capon, F., Levato, C., Bussaglia, E., Lo Cicero, S., Tizzano, E.F., Baiget, M., Silani, V., Pizzuti, A., Novelli, G. & Dallapiccola, B. (1996a): Deletion analysis of the simple tandem repeat loci physically linked to the spinal muscular atrophy locus. *Hum. Mutat.* **7,** 138–200.

Capon, F., Levato, C., Semprini, S., Pizzuti, A., Mezlini, L., Novelli, G. & Dallapiccola, B. (1996b): Deletion analysis of SMN and NAIP genes in spinal muscular atrophy Italian families. *Muscle & Nerve* **19,** 378–80.

Chasouat, G., Lochu, P., Ville, Y., Rhali, H., Bedossa, P., Selva, J., Bergere, M., D'Auriol, L., Bellet, D., Vidault, M. & Frydman, R. (1994): Transcervical sampling: a preliminary prospective study. In: *Fetal cells in maternal blood,* eds. J.L. Simpson. & S. Elias. *Ann. N. Y. Acad. Sci.* **731,** 197–200.

Collins, F. (1992): Positional cloning: let's not call it reverse any more. *Nature Genet.* **1,** 3–6.

Daniels, R.J., Thomas, N.H., MacKinnon, R.N., Lehner, T., Ott, J., Flint, T.J., Dubowitz, V., Ignatius, J., Donner, M., Zerres, K., Rietschel, M., Cookson, W.O.C., Brzustowicz, L.M., Gilliam, T.C. & Davies, K.E. (1992): Linkage analysis of spinal muscular atrophy. *Genomics* **12**, 335–339.

Gal, A., Mucke, J., Theile, H., Wieacker, P.F., H-H. & Wienker, T.F. (1985): X-linked dominant Charcot–Marie–Tooth disease: suggestion of linkage with a cloned DNA sequence from the proximal Xq. *Hum. Genet.* **70**, 38–42.

Gennarelli, M., Novelli, G., Andreasi-Bassi, F., Mardorell, L., Cornet, M., Menegazzo, E., Mostacciuolo, M.L., Martinez, J.M., Angelini, C., Pizzuti, A., Baiget, M. & Dallapiccola, B. (1996): Prediction of myotonic dystrophy clinical severity based on number of intragenic (CTG) trinucleotide repeats. *Amer. J. Med. Genet.* **65**, 342–347.

Gilliam, T.C., Brzustowicz, L.M., Castilla, L.H., Lehner, T., Penchaszadeh, G.K., Daniels, R.J., Byth B.C., Knowles, J., Hislop, J.E., Shapira, Y., Penchaszadeh, G.K., Daniels, R.J., Byth, B.C., Knowles, J., Hislop, J.E., Shapira, Y., Dubowitz, V., Munsat, T.L., Ott, J. & Davies, K.E. (1990): Genetic homogeneity between acute and chronic forms of spinal muscular atrophy. *Nature* **345**, 823–825.

Ishai, D., Amiel, A., Diukman, R., Cogan, O., Lichtenstein, Z., Abramovici, H. & Fejgin, M. (1995): Uterine cavity lavage: adding FISH to conventional cytogenetics for embryonic sexing and diagnosing common chromosomal aberrations. *Prenat. Diagn.* **15**, 961–966.

Kaplan, J.C. & Fontaine, B. (1995): Neuromuscular disorders: gene location. *Neuromusc. Disord.* **5**, 1–5.

Lefebvre, S., Burgien, L., Reboullet, S., Clermont, O., Burlet, P., Viollet, L., Benichou, B., Bruaud, C., Millasseau, P., Zeviani, M., Le Paslier, D., Frézal, J., Cohen, D., Weissenbach, J., Munnich, A. & Melchi, J. (1995): Identification and characterization of a spinal muscular atrophy-determining gene. *Cell* **80**, 1–20.

Lo Cicero, S., Capon, F., Melchionda, S., Gennarelli, M., Novelli, G. & Dallapiccola, B., (1994): First-trimester prenatal diagnosis of spinal muscular atrophy using microsatellite markers. *Prenat. Diagn.* **14**, 459–462.

Massari, A., Novelli, G., Colosimo, A., Sangiuolo, F., Palka, G., Calabrese, G., Camurri, L., Ghirardini, G., Milani, G., Giorlandino, C., Gazzanelli, G., Malatesta, M., Romanini, C. & Dallapiccola, B. (1996): Noninvasive early prenatal molecular diagnosis using retrieved transcervical trophoblast cells. *Hum. Genet.* **97**, 150–155.

Mastrogiacomo, I., Pagani, E., Novelli, G., Angelini, C., Gennarelli, M., Menegazzo, E., Bonanni, G. & Dallapiccola, B. (1994): Male hypogonadism in myotonic dystrophy is related to (CTG)n triplet mutation. *J. Endocrinol. Invest.* **17**, 381–383.

McWilliam, R.C., Gardner-Medwin, D., Doyle, D. & Stephenson, J.B.P. (1985): Diaphragmatic paralysis due to spinal muscular atrophy. An unrecognised cause of respiratory failure in infancy? *Arch. Dis. Child* **60**, 145–149.

Melacini, P., Villanova, C., Menegazzo, E., Novelli, G., Danieli, G.A., Rizzoli, G., Fasoli, G., Angelini, C., Buja, G., Miorelli, M., Dallapiccola, B. & Dalla Volta, S. (1995): Correlation between cardiac involvement and CTG trinucleotide repeat length in myotonic dystrophy. *JACC* **25**, 239–245.

Monk, M. (1992): Fetal nucleated cells in the maternal circulation. In: *Prenatal diagnosis and screening*, eds. D.J.H. Brock, C.H. Rodeck & M.A. Ferguson-Smith, pp. 627–638. London: Churchill Livingstone.

Müller, U., Graeber, M.B., Haberhausen, G. & Köhler, A. (1994): Molecular basis and diagnosis of neurogenetic disorders. *J. Neurol. Sci.* **124**, 119–140.

Novelli, G., Gennarelli, M., Fattorini, C., Abruzzese, C. & Dallapiccola, B. (1993a): The dynamic genomics of myotonic dystrophy and its clinical relevance: an overview. *Biomed. Pharmacother.* **47**, 321–330.

Novelli, G., Gennarelli, M., Menegazzo, E., Mostacciuolo, M.L., Pizzuti, A., Fattorini, C., Tessarolo, D., Tomelleri, G., Giacanelli, M., Danieli, G.A., Rizzuto, N., Caskey, C.T., Angelini, C. & Dallapiccola, B. (1993b): (CTG)n triplet mutation and phenotype manifestations in myotonic dystrophy patients. *Biochem. Med. Metab. Biol.* **50**, 85–92.

Novelli G., Capon, F., Tamisari, L., Grandi, E., Angelini, C., Guerrini, P. & Dallapiccola B. (1995a): Neonatal spinal muscular atrophy with diaphragmatic paralysis is unlinked to 5q11.2–q13. *J. Med. Genet.* **32**, 216–219.

Novelli, G., Gennarelli, M., Menegazzo, E. & Dallapiccola, B. (1995b): Discordant clinical outcome in myotonic dystrophy relatives showing (CTG)n 700 repeats. *Neuromusc. Disord.* **5**, 157–159.

Pertl, B., Davies, A., Soothill, P., Rodeck, C. & Adinolfi, M.C. (1994): Detection of fetal cells in endocervical samples. In: *Fetal cells in maternal blood*, eds J.L. Simpson & S. Elias. *Ann. N. Y. Acad. Sci.* **731**, 186–192.

Pizzuti, A., Colosimo, A., Ratti, A., Capon F., Gennarelli, M., Silani, V., Ghezzi, C., Lo Cicero, S., Calabrese, G., Palka, G.D., Scarlato, G., Novelli, G. & Dallapiccola, B. (1995): Identification of multiple transcribed sequences from the spinal muscular atrophy region on human chromosome 5. *Biochem. Biophys. Res. Commun.* **206**, 294–301.

Roy, N., Mahadevan, M.S., McLean, M., Shutler, G., Yaraghi, Z., Farahani, R., Baird, S., Besner-Johnston, A., Lefebvre, C., Kang, X., Salih, M., Aubry, H., Tamai, K., Guan, X., Ioannou, P., Crawford, T.O., de Jong, P.J., Surh, L., Ikeda J.E., Korneluk, R.G. & MacKenzie, A. (1995): The gene for neuronal apoptosis inhibitory protein is partially deleted in individuals with spinal muscular atrophy. *Cell* **80,** 167–178.

Yates, Y.R.W., Malcolm, S. & Read, A.P. (1989): Guidelines for DNA banking. *J. Med. Genet.* **26,** 245–250.

Conclusions

The provision of global care for the patient with neuromuscular disease and his family

Giovanni Lanzi

Department of Child Neuropsychiatry, C. Mondino Institute, University of Pavia, Via Palestro 3, 27100 Pavia, Italy

Summary

The paper discusses the need for neuromuscular patients to be treated globally, avoiding excessive technicality and the inevitable fragmentation of treatment among different specialists which has resulted from scientific advances. Such patients and their families need a physician who can develop an empathic relationship with them and meet their needs globally. Three critical points in the treatment of these patients are identified: (1) when a precise diagnosis is made; (2) when this is communicated; and (3) when the provision of care is made for the patient and his family. In the absence of a cure, life expectancy and quality of life are not just biological problems, but can be improved by a therapeutic alliance between the patient, the family and the physician who is truly able to support them.

Clinical and scientific interest in patients with neuromuscular diseases has grown in Italy, and elsewhere over recent years, as is shown by the number of centres and physicians who now work with them. The concept that an interdisciplinary approach to these patients' treatment is necessary has gained more and more ground, and for this reason the patients have dealings with a wide range of specialists: the child neuropsychiatrist, the neurologist, the paediatrician, the psychologist, the orthopaedist, the physiotherapist, the pneumologist, the cardiologist, the geneticist, etc.

At the same time another idea has gained ground: that although it is in general true that these patients cannot, at least for the time being, be cured, they can be treated and the physician is thus responsible for seeking every means not just to keep them alive but also to improve their quality of life.

It should be remembered that in the past, when such a diagnosis, and thus an unfavourable prognosis, was made, and when it had been established that all treatment was ineffective, the physician lost interest in these patients and left them to their fate. The situation is nowadays very different, thanks to experience gained over the last few decades in the light of new discoveries, especially in the field of genetics.

In the light of scientific developments and the current possibilities for practical intervention, the provision of care for the patient with a neuromuscular disease poses many problems to the physician on which I feel it would be useful to reflect. In this paper I shall not deal with what can be done nowadays to care for and rehabilitate these patients, since others have already dealt with the topic in depth; rather I believe it may be interesting to spend some time thinking about some general issues in care provision for such patients, given their importance if there really is a desire to meet the needs of the patient and his family.

In order that the physician can carry out his functions suitably, I think that it is necessary for him – even more today than in the past – to be prepared to approach the patient and his family in a frankly empathic way, always being ready to listen to their many needs: able to treat the physical disease, but also to understand and contain the anguish which the chronic and progressive pathology involves. It is only in this way that the physician will be able to make a response to the patient and his family which is not sectorial but is global, as the sufferer would actually need and like.

In the light of our experience in treating patients with neuromuscular pathologies, I should like to make some comments with particular reference to three phases of our work for them: (1) when a precise diagnosis is made; (2) when this is communicated; (3) when the provision for care and treatment for the patient and his family is made.

In this paper I shall make particular reference to our work with patients with Duchenne's muscular dystrophy and spinal muscular atrophy with onset in the first years of life; these are indeed the neuromuscular patients most commonly met.

Making the diagnosis

The importance of a precise diagnosis seems to be rather obvious, if it is borne in mind that it is the basis for our treatment of both the patient and the family.

Great importance must certainly be attached to the symptomatology which a child or adolescent presents, because it is most useful for formulating a reliable diagnosis and establishing what instrumental tests are necessary. It is therefore very important to gather every possible piece of clinical and anamnestic information on the patient and his family, since, as in every field of medicine, we may be sure of our diagnosis only when the laboratory findings agree with our clinical hypotheses.

The dosage of haematic enzymes like CPK, LDH and Aldolase; electromyograms and the measurement of the velocity of conduction of movement and senses; and muscle and nerve biopsies, are all certainly fundamental for an accurate diagnosis of a neuromuscular disease, but without a clinician who is competent in this field, and is therefore aware of what should be asked of these examinations, there is the risk of making an inaccurate diagnosis.

New discoveries in genetics have brought about a revolution in this field. Geneticists tell us that in a short time PCR (protein chain reaction) diagnosis should become routine, and because of the technique's relative simplicity (a small quantity of any biological material is sufficient) and its low cost it should be available to even district hospitals.

This field is in constant evolution but paradoxically we may say that genetics has changed clinical practice because it is only through a good knowledge of the clinical situation that a problem-solving use of genetic tests can be made.

This very idea was expressed by Hausmanova-Petrusewicz *et al.* (1992) in a recent article on diagnostic methods in spinal muscular atrophy. She reports that 15 per cent of her patients did not have the genetic defect in chromosome 5, so the clinician still has a definite and important role to play in this sphere.

Genetic heterogeneity is present in various neuromuscular pathologies (e.g. Charcot–Marie–Tooth polyneuropathy, in which various loci can correspond to an identical symptomatology), and conversely clinicians have long known about the clinical heterogeneity which may even be found in the same family, as in the above-mentioned Charcot–Marie–Tooth disease and in spinal muscular atrophies. Given this heterogeneity it is easy to understand why a correct diagnosis should not only be able to give a name to the disease, but also express a precise prognosis, and assess the resources available to the patient and the compensatory mechanisms which have been set in motion. It is obvious that the patient needs all these things, and expects them of us.

Our responsibilities do not finish here, if it is borne in mind that in genetic diseases the family members must be checked. There is a clear obligation to provide explanations and early preventive measures.

Communication of the diagnosis

This is certainly one of the most difficult and painful moments which we experience in our clinical practice. Whenever we have to do this, we are well aware that we shall cause a serious psychological injury in the parents, a double mourning, (1) because we are telling them that the disease from which their child is suffering will lead to death or, in the most fortunate cases, to a progressive invalidity, even if a number of years may pass; and (2) because such a disease is hereditary, and has been transmitted to the patient by them or one of them and the same could happen to any other children they might have.

For both these reasons the shock our diagnosis brings about in the parents can be well understood, and, as Lanzi *et al.* (1991) report, they remember even after many years the moment in which it was communicated to them. As a result great care and attention must clearly be dedicated to this delicate moment. Obviously, no one doubts the need to communicate a true and accurate diagnosis to the family, but it is also true that it is necessary to be very careful to choose the most suitable means and time so that the news can be absorbed as well as possible.

It is precisely for this reason that it should be borne in mind that all parents need, from the moment the diagnosis is communicated, to see a willingness in the physician who is before them to understand and share in their suffering beyond the obligation to provide some relief.

It is easy to understand why these parents initially reject the diagnosis of neuromuscular disease, especially when faced with forms with a particularly unfavourable course – a diagnosis which tragically they may sometimes suspect from various clues, be they familiar or personal, but cannot foresee when the symptoms have not yet all presented. (Sometimes such diagnoses may be made by chance, particularly with small children). They instinctively also reject the physician who makes the diagnosis, but it is precisely at this moment that the physician can show real openness, avoiding taking up rigid and dogmatic positions, even if these would be supported by undeniable technical expertise. It is not really the physician who is being rejected, but the truth he is seeking to communicate.

After the diagnosis has been communicated, the family expects that the physician will help them to gradually acknowledge the truth and in some way succeed in accepting it. At this point they often want a second opinion from other specialists or hospitals, and expect that the physician will understand this need and help them to do so correctly. It is important to grasp this need when it is expressed, and give such help to avoid the family's taking their own initiative and keeping it hidden from the physician, which for them is more difficult, painful, and usually rather inconclusive. If, on the other hand, the physician is able to grasp their need and guides them correctly, they will then really be able to feel trust and will be better able to let themselves be helped and guided. In that case that therapeutic alliance between the physician and the family can begin, which is fundamental if treatment is to be given and experienced correctly, through the various stages of the disease.

It seems right to emphasize at this point how families form a negative judgement of those physicians who, after being involved in the process of diagnosis, leave to others the job of communicating the diagnosis they have made without any further contact with them. The families justly reject this type of behaviour, since they need to discuss the diagnosis at length with the physician who has made it, expressing their doubts, their rejection, and their inability to accept it. I can only share in these expectations of the family and warn that an excessive technicality will slowly deprive the physician of any specific role, which is also that of relating to the patient and his family, answering all the patient's needs, not just those which are strictly biological.

If the physician is not able to grasp the importance of this moment and does not make allowances for all the psychological difficulties experienced by the patient and the family after the communication of such a diagnosis, it will become difficult to satisfy their needs.

So far I have spoken of the communication of the diagnosis to the family and not to the patient directly; deliberately so, since I deal with paediatric patients. The problem could, however, arise when dealing with pre-adolescents or adolescents. It is rare for sick children directly to ask the physicians who are treating them for a diagnosis and prognosis; often they prefer to have these answers from their parents, and in particular from the mother. It happens otherwise only when the physician or physiotherapist dedicates sufficient time to the patient in frequent meetings that an empathic and in-depth relationship develops between them.

Provision of care for patients and their families for treatment

I wrote above that the study and treatment of neuromuscular diseases have now become completely interdisciplinary, so that the patient ends up being treated by various specialists. We have had some quite good examples at this conference, with rich and up-to-date papers in various specific sectors of the provision of care for neuromuscular patients.

However it is precisely this interdisciplinarity, which has become progressively greater in recent years, that has ended up posing patients with new problems. They at times runs the risk of feeling that they are being treated by everybody, but by no one in a satisfying and complete way.

Patients and their families obviously do not like this pattern of medical care, and they would like, as well as refined medical care and rehabilitation, to have someone alongside them who becomes a unique point of reference for their every need. This person should be capable of co-ordinating to some extent the various interventions that are planned and carried out, taking on personally, as they do, part of the responsibility.

It is true that no physician can have sufficient expertise in all the specific fields which are involved in the care of these patients, but it is also true that patients do not want to feel themselves divided up into many separate sectors because this increases their anguish. Instead, they seek a physician who knows everything about their condition and is responsible for their daily care, so that they can be certain of being known and cared for as a complete individual.

I feel that this aspect is of fundamental importance for these patients. It is only in this way that they can identify the physician who is monitoring them as their own.

I do not feel that it can be decided *a priori* which of the various specialists involved in treating a patient should take on this role. It is for patients to choose, after having evaluated how each specialist relates to them. It is, however, important that physicians understand this need of dystrophy patients and collaborate in a concrete way, so that what I have outlined above can be achieved, without tensions or contradictions, in the sole interest of patients and their families.

The families and patients themselves feel a very real need to have someone who takes responsibility for them among the many specialists they meet, so as to establish, above all with the patient, that alliance of which I have already spoken.

We may say, within the limits of the possibilities of treating these diseases, that it is this very alliance which becomes, at a certain point of the treatment, the most important aspect of the physician's activity. When patients deteriorate, and the biological treatments show themselves more and more ineffective, the presence of the physician alongside the patients and their families may become particularly useful, if he is able to listen to and contain their ever more anguishing experiences. This presence becomes the fundamental aspect of the therapeutic alliance.

It is not only the patient who needs support at this point, but also the parents – particularly the mother, to whom the most painful aspects of the situation are often left. Thus the attending physician must above all pay particular attention to her, supporting her and helping her in the difficulties she meets.

We know how much better it is for patients, when the defences they have used up to this point are no longer sufficient and they realize that they are getting progressively worse, to find someone who is prepared to listen to their fears, rather then someone who tries to silence them.

Nowadays the problem of dying often takes physicians themselves by surprise, as they more or less unconsciously tend not only to detach themselves from it, but also to detach the problem from the individuals they are treating. In so doing, however, they do not realize and do not take into account how useful it can be for patients to have someone close to them, to whom they can communicate their fears: for silence is more difficult to bear than the reality itself.

Given the impossibility, at least for the moment, of curing these patients, it is important to make every effort to put into effect all the rehabilitative treatments which are possible today. Everything must also be done to preserve a dialogue with them and their families, because only thus is it possible for these patients to maintain their faith in the person who is treating them. These also seem to be the premisses for their continuing to hope and to make every effort to carry out the treatment which is asked of them.

References

Hausmanova-Petrusewicz, I., Zaremba, J. & Prot, G. (1992): Genetic investigations on chronic forms of infantile and juvenile spinal muscular atrophy. *Acta Cardiomyol.* **1,** 17–23.

Lanzi, G., Besana, D., Balottin, U. & Aliprandi, M.T. (1991): Relational and therapeutic aspects of children with late onset of a terminal disease. *Child's Nerv. Syst.* **9,** 339–342.

Subject Index

A

acquired autoimmune myasthenia gravis	78
acute rhabdomyolysis	3–4
age at onset	3
Alpers syndrome	16
Andersen's disease (muscular glycogenoses type IV)	2, 5, 6
atonic-sclerotic syndrome	23

B

Bannayan-Riley-Ruvalcaba syndrome	6
Barth syndrome	15–16
Becker's muscular dystrophy	32–33
carriers	34
genetic counselling	128, 129
orthopaedic treatment	89, 91
beta-oxidation defects	2
Britain	26

C

Canada	67
cardiomyopathies	2, 4–5, 6, 7, 14
dilated	14
hypertrophic	15–16
maternally inherited adult-onset	14
respiratory chain defects	15–16
carnitine cycle defects	2, 5
Caucasians	52
CDMY *see* chondrodystrophic myotonia	
central core disease	37, 38, 41–43
Charcot-Marie-Tooth disease 57–63	
1	58, 59, 60, 62
1A	57, 58, 60, 61, 62
1A-REP	60, 61
1B 5	7, 60
1C	60
2	58, 59
2A	57
clinical features	58–59
differential diagnosis	62–63
genetics	60
neurophysiological features	59
pathological features	59
polyneuropathy	147
tomaculous neuropathy	60–62
X	57, 135
chloride channel myotonias	48, 50
chondrodystrophic myotonia	48, 51
chronic inflammatory demyelinating polyradiculoneuropathies	62
CMD *see* congenital muscular dystrophies	
complex IV or cytochrome oxidase deficiency	10, 11, 12, 13, 14, 15, 16
congenital acetylcholine receptor deficiency	85
congenital anomalies with polycystic kidney	2
congenital fibre type disproportion	43
congenital muscular dystrophies	23–27, 43
congenital myasthenic syndromes	78, 81–85
congenital myopathies	37–44, 97, 126
central core disease	41–43
dystrophic type	38, 43–44
myotubular/centronuclear	38–40, 42
nemaline	38, 40–41, 42
congenital myotonic dystrophy	51, 53, 89, 139, 140
contractures	90–91
Cori's disease (muscular glycogenoses type III)	1–2, 4, 5, 7
COX *see* complex IV or cytochrome oxidase	

D

De Toni-Debre-Fanconi syndrome	15
Déjérine-Sottas disease *see* Charcot-Marie-Tooth disease 1	
dentatorubro-pallidoluysian atrophy	51
diagnosis	146–148
distal dystrophy	89
dominant congenital myotonia	50
Duchenne's muscular dystrophy	27, 31–32
carriers	34, 35
genetic counselling	128
global care provision	146
mechanical ventilation	104–111
orthopaedic treatment	89, 90, 91
and scoliosis	97
see also home mechanical ventilation	
dystrophic myotonic syndromes	51
dystrophies	
distal	89
Emery-Dreifuss	89, 91
oculopharyngeal	89
Steinert's	105
see also muscular	
dystrophinopathies	31–35, 129
Becker's muscular dystrophy	32–34
cardiac involvement	34–35
Duchenne's muscular dystrophy	31–32, 34, 35
unusual forms	33–34

E

Ekbom syndrome	13
electrophysiological examinations	4
Emery-Dreifuss dystrophy	89, 91
encephalomyopathies	6, 16
end-plate acetylcholinesterase deficiency	84–85
exercise intolerance	3

F

facioscapulohumeral muscular dystrophy	89, 90
familial infantile myasthenia	83–84
family history	3
fasting intolerance	3
fatiguability, abnormal	4
fatty acid transport and oxidation effects	2
FCMD *see* Fukuyama congenital muscular dystrophy	
Finland	23, 24
forearm ischaemic exercise test	4
fractures	92–93
fragile X syndrome	51, 52
France	67, 113–120
Friedreich's ataxia	13, 97–98
Fukuyama congenital muscular dystrophy	23, 24, 27, 43

G

genetic counselling	123–130
Germany	123
global care provision	145–149
diagnosis	146–148
provision of care	148–149
GSD *see* muscular glycogenoses	

H

Haw River syndrome	51
heartbeat disorders	5
hereditary motor and sensory neuropathy *see* Charcot-Marie-Tooth disease	
hereditary neuralgic amyotrophy	61
hereditary neuropathy with liability to pressure palsies *see* tomaculous neuropathy	
hereditary paraplegias	127
hereditary myotonic syndromes	47–53
calcium channel disorders	50–51
chloride channel disorders	48, 50
dystrophic	51
myotonic dystrophy	51–53
non-dystrophic myotonias	48–49
sodium channel myotonias	48, 49
hip dislocation	92
home mechanical ventilation and Duchenne's muscular dystrophy	113–120
imperative ventilation	116–118
literature review	114–115
multicentric group evaluation of techniques	115
preventive ventilation	118–120
Huntington disease	51
hyperkalaemic periodic paralysis	49
hyperlactacidaemia	5
hypokalaemic periodic paralysis	50–51

I

infantile botulism	78, 86
intergenomic communication defects	14–15
intergenomic signalling defects	2
ion channel diseases	126
see also hereditary myotonic syndromes	
isolated proximal myopathy	13
Italy	81, 140, 145

J

Japan	23–24, 52
juvenile myasthenia gravis	78, 79–81

Subject Index

K

Kearns-Sayre syndrome	5, 7, 13–14
Kennedy's disease	51
ketoacidosis	5
Krabbe's universal muscle hypoplasia	41
KSS *see* Kearns-Sayre syndrome	
Kugelberg-Welander disease	73

L

Lambert-Eaton myasthenic syndrome	77, 78, 85–86
Leber hereditary optic neuropathy	11, 14
Leigh syndrome	11, 13, 16
maternally inherited	14
lesions	96
limb-girdle muscular dystrophy	89, 90, 91, 129
lipid storage myopathy	2
liver dysfunction	5

M

McArdle's disease (muscular glycogenoses type V)	2, 3, 4, 6
Machado-Joseph disease	51
maternally inherited Leigh syndrome	14
MEB *see* muscle-eye-brain disease	
mechanical ventilation	103–111
Duchenne's muscular dystrophy	104–111
pathophysiological bases	104–108
sleep-disordered breathing	109–110
see also home	
MELAS *see* mitochondrial encephalomyopathy with lactic acidosis and stroke-like episodes	
mental retardation syndrome with fragile X type E	51
merosin non-deficient congenital muscular dystrophies	26, 27
merosin-deficient congenital muscular dystrophies	26
MERRF *see* myoclonus epilepsy and ragged red fibres	
metabolic myopathies	1–7, 126
clinical approach	3–7
minicore disease	38, 42–43
mitochondrial diseases	2
mitochondrial DNA	2, 9, 10, 11–14, 16
mitochondrial encephalomyopathy with lactic acidosis and stroke-like episodes	7, 12, 13, 14
mitochondrial neurogastrointestinal encephalopathy	15
molecular prenatal diagnosis	131–142
approaches	134
Charcot-Marie-Tooth disease	135
human gene map	132
NAIP gene	139
personal experience	141
SMA	136, 138, 139
SMA I	137, 138, 139
motoneurone	96
mtDNA *see* mitochondrial	
multicore disease	42–43
muscle-eye-brain disease	24, 43
muscular dystrophies	126
congenital	23–27, 43
facioscapulohumeral	89, 90
limb-girdle	89, 90, 91, 129
orthopaedic treatment	89–93
contractures	90–91
fractures	92–93
hip dislocation	92
orthopaedic management	90
scoliosis	92
see also Becker's; Duchenne's	
muscular findings	3
muscular glycogenoses (GSD)	1–2
type II (Pompe's disease)	1, 3, 5, 6
type III (Cori's disease)	1–2, 4, 5, 7
type IV (Andersen's disease)	2, 5, 6
type V (McArdle's disease)	2, 3, 4, 6
type VII (Tarui's disease)	2, 4, 6
muscular lesions	96
muscular symptoms	4
muscular weakness, fluctuating	4
myasthenia	
familial infantile	83–84
penicillamine-induced	78, 86
myasthenia gravis	81
acquired auto immune	78
juvenile	78, 79–81
transient neonatal	78–79
myasthenic syndromes	77
congenital	78, 81–85
Lambert-Eaton	77, 78, 85–86
myoclonus epilepsy and ragged-red fibres	7, 13, 14
myopathies	15
isolated proximal	13
lipid storage	2
metabolic	1–7, 126
myotubular/centronuclear	38–40, 42
nemaline	40–41, 42, 88
quadriceps	34
see also cardiomyopathies; congenital	
myotonia	47, 49
chloride channel	48, 50
chondrodystrophic	48, 51
non-dystrophic	48–49
paradoxical	47, 49
recessive generalized	50
sodium channel	48, 49
see also hereditary	
myotonic dystrophy	47, 48, 51–53, 128, 139, 140
clinical-genetic relationships	52–53
dominant congenital	50
gene, molecular biology of	51–52
mutation mechanism	52
prenatal diagnosis	141
see also congenital	
myotonic syndromes	126
dystrophic	51
see also hereditary	
myotubular/centronuclear myopathy	38–40, 42

153

N

nDNA *see* nuclear	
nemaline myopathy	38, 40–41, 42
nerve lesions, peripheral	96
neurogenic atrophy, ataxia, retinitis pigmentosa	11, 14
neurogenic muscular atrophy	138
neurogenic syndromes	127
neuromuscular junction	77, 78, 79
neuromuscular transmission disorders in childhood	77–86
acquired autoimmune myasthenia gravis	78
congenital myasthenic syndromes	78, 81–85
infantile botulism	78, 86
juvenile myasthenia gravis	78, 79–81
Lambert-Eaton myasthenic syndrome	77, 78, 85–86
penicillamine-induced myasthenia gravis	78, 86
transient neonatal myasthenia gravis	78–79
non-dystrophic myotonias	48–49
nuclear DNA	2, 9, 10, 11, 15

O

oculopharyngeal dystrophy	89

P

paradoxical myotonia	47, 49
paramyotonia congenita	49
Pearson syndrome	13–14
penicillamine-induced myasthenia gravis	78, 86
PEO *see* progressive external opthalmoplegia	
Pompe's disease (muscular glycogenoses type II)	1, 3, 5, 6
progressive external opthalmoplegia	7, 10, 12, 13–14
provocation tests	4
purine metabolism anomaly	2

Q

quadriceps myopathy	34

R

ragged-red fibres	11, 12, 13, 14, 15, 16
Ramsey Hunt syndrome	13
recessive generalized myotonia	50
respiration *see* mechanical ventilation	
respiratory chain defects	9–16
cardiomyopathies	15–16
clinical syndromes associated with mtDNA defects	11–14
clinical syndromes with intergenomic communication defects	14–15
clinical syndromes with probable nDNA defects	15
encephalomyopathies	16
morphological criteria	11
myopathies	15
Rett syndrome	98
Reye's syndrome	2, 6
rigid spine syndromes	23

S

scapuloperoneal dystrophy	89
scoliosis	92, 95–101
causes of deformities	96–97
surgical indications and techniques	100–101
treatment decisions	98–100
types of deformities	97–98
Sengers syndrome	16
SIDS *see* sudden infant death syndrome	
slow channel syndrome	85
sodium channel myotonias	48, 49
Spain	140
spinal muscular atrophy	67–74, 97, 128, 136, 137, 138, 139, 146, 147
classification	68–69
definitions	69
I	70–71, 72, 74, 137, 138, 139
II	72–73, 74
III	72, 73, 74
intermediate	71
mild	73
recent advances	67–68
severe	69
spinocerebellar ataxia type 1	51, 52
Steinert's dystrophy	105
sudden infant death syndrome	2, 5, 6

T

Tarui's disease (muscular glycogenoses VII)	2, 4, 6
tomaculous neuropathy	57, 60–62, 63
transient neonatal myasthenia gravis	78–79
Turkey	26
type I fibre predominance	42–43

U

United States	123

V

ventilation *see* home; mechanical

W

Walker-Warburg syndrome	23, 24, 43
Werdnig-Hoffmann disease	69